Psycho-pharmacology Consultation

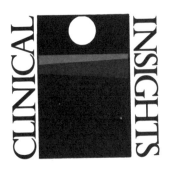

CLINICAL INSIGHTS

Psycho-pharmacology Consultation

Edited by
DAVID C. JIMERSON, M.D.

Chief, Section on Biomedical Psychiatry, Laboratory of Clinical Science, National Institute of Mental Health

JOHN P. DOCHERTY, M.D.

Medical Director, Nashua Brookside Hospital

AMERICAN PSYCHIATRIC PRESS, INC.
Washington, D.C.

Copyright © 1986 American Psychiatric Press, Inc.

ALL RIGHTS RESERVED

Manufactured in the U.S.A.

The paper used in this publication meets the minimum requirements of American National Standard for Information Sciences–Permanence of Paper for Printed Library Materials, ANSI Z39.48-1984. ∞™

Library of Congress Cataloging in Publication Data

Main entry under title.

Psychopharmacology consultation.

(Clinical insights)
Updated and expanded version of material presented at a symposium at the annual meeting of the American Psychiatric Association, May 1984.
Includes bibliographies.
1. Psychopharmacology consultation—Congresses. I. Jimerson, David C., 1946–   . II. Docherty, John P., 1944–   . III. American Psychiatric Association. Meeting (137th: 1984: Los Angeles, Calif.) IV. Series. [DNLM: 1. Mental Disorders—drug therapy—congresses. 2. Referral and Consultation—congresses. WM 402 P974]
RC483.3.P78   1986   616.89'18   86-14136
ISBN 0-88048-141-2 (soft)

Contents

Contributors

JOHN P. DOCHERTY, M.D.
Medical Director, Nashua Brookside Hospital, Nashua, New Hampshire

ROBERT H. GERNER, M.D.
Associate Professor, Neuropsychiatric Institute, University of California,
Los Angeles; Brentwood Division, West Los Angeles Veterans Administration
Medical Center; Director, Center for Mood Disorders, West Los Angeles

FREDERICK K. GOODWIN, M.D.
Director of Intramural Research, National Institute of Mental Health,
Bethesda, Maryland

DAVID C. JIMERSON, M.D.
Chief, Section on Biomedical Psychiatry, Laboratory of Clinical Science,
National Institute of Mental Health, Bethesda, Maryland

DAVID PICKAR, M.D.
Chief, Section on Clinical Studies, Clinical Neurosciences Branch,
National Institute of Mental Health, Bethesda, Maryland

EDWARD L. SCHARFMAN, M.D.
Assistant Professor of Psychiatry, New York Medical College
Psychiatric Institute, Valhalla, New York

Introduction

Consultation in psychopharmacology is an area of increasing importance in the treatment of patients with major psychiatric disorders. The evolution of clinical psychopharmacology as a subspecialty reflects in part the increasing range of clinical syndromes demonstrated to benefit from psychopharmacological treatment. There is also increasing information on new approaches for working with patients who do not respond to the customary first-line psychopharmacological interventions. New information brings new complexity, and thus the psychopharmacological consultant becomes an important resource to the eclectically trained psychiatrist who may not have an active working familiarity with recent developments in psychopharmacological research. Similarly, the psychopharmacology consultant is an important resource for nonphysician psychotherapists and nonpsychiatric physicians who have questions about the appropriateness or potential complications of using psychopharmacological agents with a particular patient.

In this monograph we highlight new developments in selected clinical settings encountered by the psychopharmacology consultant. In Chapters 1 and 4, Drs. Frederick Goodwin and David Pickar outline newer strategies for confronting problems in the psychopharmacological management of major depressive illness and schizophrenia, respectively. Dr. Robert Gerner and I (D.J.) review studies in Chapters 2 and 3 that provide evidence for the efficacy of psychopharmacological approaches in patients with anxiety syndromes and eating disorders, respectively. Dr. Edward Scharfman describes the role of the psychopharmacology consultant in the general hospital and presents several clinical vignettes in Chapter 5. Then, to end the monograph, I (J.D.) remind readers of a range of important psychosocial issues to consider in the psychopharmacological treatment of psychiatric patients.

This monograph is an updated and expanded version of material presented in a symposium at the 1984 annual meeting of the American Psychiatric Association. Dr. Richard Shader's contribution to that symposium as discussant is gratefully acknowledged, particularly because a number of his suggestions have been incorporated into these chapters.

David C. Jimerson, M.D.
John P. Docherty, M.D.

Pharmacological Consultation in Major Depressive Disorders

Frederick K. Goodwin, M.D.

1

Pharmacological Consultation in Major Depressive Disorders

A physician has many options when faced with a complex psychopharmacology consultation. To present them in this chapter, I melded information from the research literature and from clinical experience. Although the focus is on six types of clinical problems common in psychopharmacology consultation of patients with major depressive illness (see Table 1), many of the principles apply to psychopharmacology consultation for patients with other psychiatric disorders. My intention is to pragmatically address common clinical problems and not to detail the extensive research literature supporting many of the recommendations offered.

CLINICAL EVALUATION OF ANTIDEPRESSANT-NONRESPONSIVE PATIENTS

Perhaps the most common problem in psychopharmacology consultation of major depressive disorders is nonresponse of a depressed patient to trials with two or more tricyclic or heterocyclic antidepressants. What should the consultant do in this situation? The first and most important step is to reevaluate the patient's

This research was performed by the author in his capacity as an employee of the National Institute of Mental Health and is in the public domain.

Table 1. Common Clinical Problems in Psychopharmacology Consultation of Major Depressive Disorders

Problem
Poor clinical response to a tricyclic or heterocyclic antidepressant drug
Pharmacological approaches to treatment of a borderline patient with severe mood lability and episodic dyscontrol
Symptomatic relapse following initial response to a tricyclic antidepressant drug
Breakthrough depression during lithium treatment in a patient with bipolar disorder
Poor treatment response in a rapidly cycling bipolar patient
Management of side effects of antidepressant drugs

diagnosis and clinical state, because a great majority of the difficulties associated with the drug treatment of depression are due to lack of diagnostic precision. We have been helped considerably in recent years by the evolution of the *Diagnostic and Statistical Manual of Mental Disorders (Third Edition)* (DSM-III; American Psychiatric Association 1980) criteria. Diagnosis of the affective and other psychiatric disorders no longer must depend on one's etiologic point of view but rather can be linked to reliable and consistent descriptors of behavior. Although no fixed set of criteria can adequately match the complex process of pattern recognition used by the experienced diagnostician, standardized criteria combined with clinical experience can make the diagnostic process more intelligible. The most definitive descriptor of a major depressive episode is dysphoric mood, followed by a cluster of other symptoms. At least five of these symptoms are required, including disturbances of appetite and sleep regulation, loss of energy, psychomotor retardation or agitation, various mood changes, loss of interest, slowed thinking (a very important and often undervalued symptom in serious depression), self-blame or inappropriate guilt, recurrent thoughts of death or suicide, and major impairment in normal role functioning. The episode must last at least 2 weeks;

however, when considering drug treatment, most clinicians would probably require an episode to have lasted at least 3–4 weeks. The further a patient departs from these typical features, the more difficult and unpredictable pharmacological management will be.

Another diagnosis problem is the underdiagnosis of bipolar disorder: Missing this diagnosis often results in inappropriate treatment requiring subsequent consultation. Textbooks tend to assign bipolar illness relatively rare status—approximately 10 percent of all affective illness. In fact, if you include in the bipolar total the group of patients who have hypomania (which is clearly a pathological state but not severe enough to require hospitalization), then the bipolar segment of major affective disorder constitutes approximately 30 percent of the whole (Krauthammer and Klerman 1979). It is simply folly to try to get a good past history of hypomania from a depressed patient. At this point convergence of information from family members and other people in the patient's life is necessary. Depressed patients often do not remember their hypomania as anything other than their good times. In any patient who presents with a history of several depressive episodes it is particularly important to pursue a history of hypomania. This is especially important if the first major depressive episode occurred before the age of 35—that is, if the age of onset is in the bipolar range. The consultant needs to ask about times of decreased need for sleep, more energy than usual, increased self-esteem, increased productivity with vigorous working hours, unusual creative thinking, uninhibited people seeking, extreme gregariousness, hypersexual behavior (often without recognition of the painful consequences), excessive involvement in pleasurable activities with a lack of concern for their consequences (particularly buying sprees, foolish business investments, or reckless driving), physical restlessness, and more talkativeness than usual. Considered in isolation, each of these symptoms seems to reflect characteristics that most of us would not mind having, at least in modest doses. Yet their implication becomes more serious when one realizes that the consequences can be painful and that this state can evolve into more serious bipolar illness, at times as a consequence of some inappropriate treatments (Akiskal 1980).

After proper diagnosis is established, what is the first step in working with a unipolar patient showing poor response to antidepressant medication? Before switching to another drug, it is critical to evaluate some basic treatment issues that are often overlooked. The first of these is poor compliance (or adherence)—one of the major problems limiting the efficacy of any drug. Estimates of noncompliance in general medicine have been as high as 50 percent. A recent survey by Jamison et al. (1979) indicates that nearly 50 percent of patients in a lithium clinic reported noncompliance at some point, and these data were from a clinic that is probably better structured than many individual practices. A second problem is excessive alcohol intake. Clinical experience suggests that chronic excessive alcohol consumption can limit the efficacy of antidepressant drugs. Some patients inadvertently increase their alcohol intake when on a drug because they are not getting quite the same effect from the alcohol. Marijuana is also a probable factor limiting tricyclic efficacy, especially its regular and heavy use. Another common limiting factor is an inappropriate blood level (American Psychiatric Association Task Force on the Use of Laboratory Tests in Psychiatry 1985). Today, reliable assays are available for most of the commonly prescribed drugs, but one still must be cautious. It is useful to ask commercial laboratories for their reference standards and a description of the assay methodology. In addition, it can be revealing to send a few blinded duplicate samples as a periodic check.

Alternative Medication Strategies for Nonresponders

After the possible role of basic treatment issues has been evaluated, the second step with the tricyclic nonresponder is to change to another tricyclic (or heterocyclic) with a different "neurotransmitter profile." Nobody knows for sure whether the difference in neurotransmitter profile accounts for the difference in antidepressant efficacy, but experienced clinicians know that, for example, some people do not respond to amitriptyline (a more serotonergic drug) and do respond to imipramine or desmethylimipramine (more noradrenergic drugs) and vice versa (Cowdry and Goodwin

1981). When making these changes, one can shift immediately to the equivalent dose of the second drug because there is cross-tolerance to the anticholinergic effects.

The proper role of the second generation antidepressants is not yet well established. Some have suggested that nonresponders to classic tricyclics deserve a trial with a second generation drug before going on to other approaches (Rudorfer et al. 1984). Also, second generation drugs can be used to take advantage of different side-effect profiles. Bupropion, a dopamine active drug, was of special interest in this case because it had virtually none of the classic anticholinergic side effects of antidepressants and was not associated with weight gain (Feighner et al. 1984).

The third step is to consider endocrine potentiation. One should evaluate thyroid function with laboratory tests—usually a T_4 and thyroid-stimulating hormone level. Unless the thyroid function is abnormally high, my own practice (particularly with female patients) is to attempt potentiation with a small amount of triiodothyronine (T_3) (25 μg is usually sufficient; some patients will respond to even half that). Although many antidepressant nonresponders will not benefit from the addition of thyroid, a patient should not be declared tricyclic resistant until after a brief (5–7 day) trial with thyroid potentiation (Goodwin et al. 1982). The potentiation of antidepressants with estrogen has also been reported (Oppenheim 1983) and may be most appropriate in post- or perimenopausal women or those who have had a total hysterectomy. Endocrine potentiation should not be prolonged; in the absence of a response, a 1- or 2-week trial is sufficient. If the patient responds, the thyroid or estrogen can be gradually withdrawn as the antidepressant dose is reduced to a maintenance level for continuation therapy (usually 9–12 months in a unipolar patient).

The next step one can take when faced with a nonresponding patient is to add lithium to the tricyclic. I list this before the monoamine oxidase inhibitors (MAOIs) simply because it can be evaluated quickly and, if not helpful, withdrawn with no complications. It has been reported that up to 60 percent of patients still unresponsive after adequate doses of tricyclics for at least 3 weeks can be converted to responders within 7–10 days after the addition of lithium carbonate at doses of 900 mg/day (De Montigny et al. 1981; Heninger et al. 1983). This strategy is based on a concept of increasing the sensitivity of some neurotransmitter receptors, although an alternative explanation is that lithium potentiation is occurring in patients who would have been lithium responsive in the first place; some of the more recurrent forms of unipolar depression respond to lithium alone (Goodwin et al. 1969). How long to continue lithium started in this way is not always clear. If the ion has indeed served primarily to potentiate the tricyclic then it could slowly be withdrawn over several weeks. If, on the other hand, one has uncovered a lithium-responsive patient, a longer treatment period might be indicated.

The next step in approaching the unipolar nonresponsive patient involves using a MAOI. In general, the MAOIs tend to be underutilized, perhaps principally because of exaggerated fears of hypertensive crises. Probably the most frequent reason clinicians use MAOIs is a patient's failure to respond to a tricyclic antidepressant (after appropriate potentiation).

A brief comment on the more primary indications for the use of MAOIs: The most frequently cited indication is a depression characterized by hypersomnia (that is, excessive sleep, albeit of diminished quality), increased appetite, and severe anergy, symptoms that are, in a sense, opposite to the classic picture of insomnia, weight loss, and appetite loss. Patients who have this cluster of symptoms might well be tried on MAOIs even before a tricyclic is tried. Another frequently cited indication for a MAOI is the presence of "atypical" depression with prominence of phobic features, hypochondriasis, and anxiety.

Another important indication for a MAOI is the treatment of bipolar patients experiencing breakthrough depressions. It is unclear whether tricyclics or MAOIs are preferable in this situation, and controlled studies are very much needed. My own preference is to treat breakthrough depressions of moderate severity with a MAOI, reserving the tricyclic for the more severe depressions, particularly those with melancholia and/or psychotic features. I return to the management of breakthrough depressions in a later section.

One additional approach to the treatment of nonresponders is the use of a MAOI/tricyclic combination. The safety of such combinations, when used appropriately, has been reviewed extensively and authoritatively by White and Simpson (1981). Clinical experience suggests that some patients who did not respond to either class of drugs alone will respond to this combination. There are two other advantages to the combination: The tricyclic given at bedtime can reduce or prevent the insomnia that often becomes the major troublesome side effect of MAOIs, and the combination may reduce the risk of the tyramine reactions to MAOIs—perhaps by inhibiting tyramine uptake into the nerve ending and therefore reducing its access to MAO (Kline et al. 1981); however, more recent data do not support this conclusion (Abrams et al. 1985; Pare et al. 1985). When using the combination of a MAOI and a tricyclic antidepressant, one must be very cautious about the sequence, and either start the two drugs together or the tricyclic first. If one starts the MAOI first, a hypertensive reaction could be produced by the subsequent addition of the tricyclic. Both drugs should be started at low doses and increased gradually to a therapeutic dose approximately half that needed when each drug is used individually. It is best to give the MAOI early in the day and the tricyclic at bedtime.

Other treatments may be considered for patients who do not respond to other pharmacological treatments. These include electroconvulsive therapy, stimulants, sleep deprivation, and various other supplements, including amino acids. The use of high-intensity light treatment for patients with seasonal depression (Rosenthal et al. 1985) is a separate issue that, unfortunately, cannot be covered because of lack of space.

DEPRESSION IN BORDERLINE PATIENTS

A most difficult problem encountered by the pharmacological consultant is the treatment of borderline patients with severe mood lability and episodic dyscontrol. The *DSM-III* criteria for borderline disorder remind us of how much of this syndrome is characterized by mood instability. Impulsivity and poorly controlled aggressive outbursts are common, and it is important not to miss the fundamental affective component in many of these patients defined as borderline. Because of the episodic nature of affective symptoms in these patients, lithium is the first alternative to consider. The MAOIs may also be helpful. Lithium and MAOIs are safe and easy to use in combination and seem to potentiate each other. In some patients, carbamazepine deserves a trial. Bupropion, a nontricyclic antidepressant that affects dopamine systems, appeared to have some promise in early experience with this particular group. Some evidence suggests that minor tranquilizers and alprazolam may exacerbate dyscontrol symptoms in some of these patients (Gardner and Cowdry 1985).

RELAPSE DURING ANTIDEPRESSANT TREATMENT

Another major, and not uncommon, problem the consultant encounters is the patient who responds to antidepressant treatment and then relapses while still on the drug. First, one should evaluate whether compliance problems or other psychosocial difficulties have occurred. Appropriate psychotherapeutic intervention may be sufficient to reestablish clinical response. Pharmacologically, one easy initial step would be to make a dose adjustment—abruptly decrease the dose by half for 1 or 2 days, then resume it at or just above the previous level. Although there are no controlled data on this, it appears to be effective about half the time, perhaps by producing a perturbation that conceivably affects receptor sensitivity. Next, one should consider the possibility that cycle induction by the original drug might explain the relapse. It is known that antidepressants can shorten the cycle length in bipolar patients (that is, decrease the time between episodes) (Wehr and Goodwin 1979). Can this effect also occur in recurrent unipolar depression? In other words, can the relapse occur for some patients because of the drug, rather than despite it? Some preliminary data suggest that cycle induction may occur in recurrent unipolar patients; at any rate the prophylactic response to lithium among this group (Schou 1979) suggests some fundamental similarities to bipolar disorder. This possibility might be kept in mind especially when a unipolar patient has an early age of onset and/or a family history of mania.

BREAKTHROUGH DEPRESSION DURING LITHIUM TREATMENT

Another frequent problem addressed by the psychopharmacological consultant is a breakthrough depression, one of the most important challenges in the management of bipolar patients on lithium. (Breakthrough manic episodes are less common and are not included here because of space limitations.) The first response to the appearance of depressive symptoms should include a reassessment of the patient's life situation with particular reference to real or perceived losses, along with a reevaluation of the lithium level. Dunner et al. (1977) showed that from 40 to 60 percent of patients having breakthrough depressions on lithium respond when the blood lithium levels are raised to 1.2 or 1.4 mEq/l. Also, A. Coppen recently reported (personal communication, 1985) that for many unipolar patients, a decrease in the lithium dose can be associated with clinical improvement.

The next step is to evaluate the possibility that lithium-induced subclinical hypothyroidism may be responsible for a breakthrough depression of moderate severity. What is the incidence of lithium-induced hypothyroidism? Using the stringent criteria familiar to endocrinology, the incidence is only 5–7 percent, but if single abnormal thyroid values are considered, the incidence approaches 20 percent. Fairly extensive clinical experience now suggests that a substantial proportion of patients with breakthrough depressions—particularly if the depression is characterized by moderate psychomotor retardation, fatigue, and hypothyroid-like symptoms—respond to supplemental thyroid. Rapid cyclers seem to be particularly vulnerable to the antithyroid effects of lithium, a finding that may relate to the relatively low efficacy of this drug in these patients.

If the response to lithium optimization and increased thyroid is not satisfactory, the clinician and patient must decide whether or not to add an antidepressant drug. If the depression is only moderately severe, it might be better to provide more psychological support and avoid antidepressants because of their potential for worsening the course of the illness. This conservative approach is especially worthwhile when the patient has been on lithium for only a year or two, as the prophylactic efficacy of lithium tends to improve with time.

On the other hand, if the depression is severe enough to cause considerable suffering and especially if normal functioning becomes significantly impaired, antidepressants are indicated. Tricyclics are still the most frequently used drugs in this situation. Among them, those with less sedative effect (such as imipramine, desmethylimipramine, or nortriptyline) are preferred, because breakthrough depressions in bipolar patients are frequently characterized by anergy and lassitude, whereas anxiety, sleep disturbance, and psychic pain are not as prominent. One of the second generation heterocyclic antidepressants may also be considered, especially if one is concerned about the greater likelihood of side effects with the traditional tricyclic drugs. On the other hand, the efficacy of these new drugs is generally not as well established, especially when the breakthrough depression is quite severe. Doses of the antidepressant should generally be somewhat lower than those used in the absence of lithium, because some side effects, such as tremor and sedation, can be additive. Because of the risk of precipitating mania/hypomania (even in the presence of lithium), these drugs should be gradually withdrawn shortly after the antidepressant response is achieved.

As noted earlier, the use of MAOIs has recently undergone somewhat of a renaissance and they are increasingly used as an alternative to tricyclic (or heterocyclic) antidepressants for the treatment of breakthrough depressions in patients on lithium. In fact, some authorities now recommend MAOIs as the treatment of choice in such cases. In a survey of lithium clinics (Gitlin et al. 1984), MAOIs were used to treat breakthrough depressions in 16 percent of the patients and tricyclics were used in 25 percent.

PHARMACOLOGICAL APPROACHES FOR RAPIDLY CYCLING BIPOLAR PATIENTS

Another problem facing the consultant is what to do with the rapidly cycling bipolar patient, that is, the individual with four or more episodes per year. Such patients are generally resistant to lithium and represent major therapeutic challenges. Dunner

(Dunner et al. 1977) has shown, in rapidly cycling patients who are not responding to lithium, that if he could maintain the lithium (that is, "tough it out") gradually over 1 or 2 years, the proportion of time the patients spent depressed and manic decreased substantially. Before he tried this he was making the problem worse (as we all have done) by precipitating manias with tricyclics and depressions with neuroleptics. Thus, the first step in managing patients who have a poor prophylactic response to lithium is to eliminate the cycle-inducing drugs, if possible.

A recent major advance in the treatment of this difficult group of patients is the anticonvulsant carbamazepine. Although some manic–depressive patients may actually show evidence of subtle temporal lobe seizures, the prophylactic efficacy of carbamazepine does not depend on electroencephalogram evidence of such seizures. The potential for bone marrow suppression by carbamazepine was overestimated earlier; it is now clear that its interaction with other anticonvulsants caused the high incidence of hematopoietic effects. Although transitory suppression of platelets is observed not infrequently, true aplastic anemia is quite rare (Post et al. 1984). In the National Institute of Mental Health (NIMH) series, about 60 percent of the rapid cyclers who had not responded to lithium showed a favorable prophylactic response after the addition of carbamazepine (Post 1985). For most patients the combination of lithium and carbamazepine seemed superior to either drug alone, although more research is urgently needed on this important question.

There is evidence that rapid cyclers have a very high incidence of diminished thyroid function (Cowdry et al. 1983), and Stancer and Persad (1982) reported successful treatment with suppressive doses of thyroid hormones. Although such an approach is not recommended for routine use in a practice, it is advisable to pay special attention to thyroid function in this group of patients and to optimize it with supplemental thyroxine whenever necessary.

SIDE EFFECTS DURING ANTIDEPRESSANT TREATMENT

The psychopharmacology consultant is often called on to help manage drug side effects. Anticholinergic side effects such as dry mouth and constipation can often be reduced by switching to a newer antidepressant with less blockade of cholinergic receptors. Excessive sedation can usually be managed by altering dosage schedules or switching to a more alerting medication. Antidepressant-induced weight gain can also be a major problem. The first approach is dietary assessment and carbohydrate restriction. The use of *l*-glutamine or tryptophan potentiation may be helpful. The tendency to produce weight gain seems to vary for different antidepressants. Thus, desipramine seems to have less tendency to cause weight gain than amitriptyline. Among the MAOIs, isocarboxazid is less likely to cause weight gain than tranylcypromine or phenelzine. One of the second generation antidepressants—bupropion—was of special interest here because it was reported to produce weight loss rather than gain (Feighner et al. 1984).

PHYSIOLOGICAL (BUT NONPHARMACOLOGICAL) TREATMENTS

Two recently developed nonpharmacological approaches to the treatment of depression (partial sleep deprivation and sleep phase advance) deserve special consideration in light of the fact that some subgroups of manic–depressive patients may be especially vulnerable to negative drug effects. The initial reports of total sleep deprivation noted dramatic but transient improvement in severe depression after one night of this procedure. In these studies an average of 75 percent of the patients experienced some amelioration of depressive symptoms on the day after sleep deprivation, the improvement generally increasing as the day went on. The beneficial effect was noted more consistently in patients with endogenous symptoms. For the great majority of patients the improvement was transient, with the depressive syndrome reappearing after the next night of sleep. A review of the major studies on the effects of total sleep deprivation suggested that, on average, 58 percent of the patients showed improvement (Gillin 1983). The improvement can apparently last more than 1 day in some of the patients.

Schilgen and Tolle (1980) evaluated the effects of sleep deprivation during the second half of the night—that is, partial sleep deprivation. Curiously, the patients in this study were put to sleep early, at 9:00 p.m., and slept until 1:00 a.m., when they were awakened. Thus, in actuality, the timing of their sleep was advanced in addition to being shortened. They studied 59 patients with endogenous depression—30 with partial sleep deprivation and 29 with total sleep deprivation. No significant differences were found between the two treatments: Both reduced depressive symptoms approximately one-third; 75 percent of the patients in both groups showed some improvement. As with the earlier reports, sleep deprivation was more effective in those patients showing clear endogenous symptoms, particularly sleep disturbance and diurnal variation. The extent to which bipolar patients were included in these studies is not specified.

In an interesting elaboration of this paradigm, our team at the NIMH (Wehr et al. 1979) treated hospitalized depressed patients with a technique that involved altering the sleep–wake cycle (phase advance). After 1 night of sleep deprivation these subjects had their sleep–wake cycles advanced 6 hrs by going to bed at 5:00 p.m. or 6:00 p.m. For the next 2 weeks they were kept on this schedule, sleeping from approximately 6:00 p.m. to 1:00 a.m. The total amount of sleep was not shortened. Sixty percent of the patients experienced rapid relief of their severe depressive symptoms and this remission persisted for approximately 2 weeks. Recently, we have enlarged this approach, applying the phase-advance technique to patients who have not responded to antidepressants (Sack et al. 1985). The phase manipulation is accomplished while the patient remains on the antidepressant drug, and the preliminary results have been encouraging.

SUMMARY

An ordered hierarchy of strategies exists for approaching the treatment-resistant depressed patient. It is important to evaluate issues such as inadequate medication dose or poor patient compliance with medication schedules before simply changing to a new drug. New strategies offer substantial promise in treating depressed patients who do not respond to an initial trial with a traditional antidepressant drug.

REFERENCES

Abrams JH, Schulman P, White WB: Successful treatment of a monooxidase inhibitor tyramine hypertensive emergency with intravenous labetolol. New Eng J Med 313:52, 1985

Akiskal HS: External validating criteria for psychiatric diagnosis: Their application in affective disorders. J Clin Psychiatry 41:6–15, 1980

American Psychiatric Association Task Force on the Use of Laboratory Tests in Psychiatry: Tricyclic antidepressants, blood level measurements and clinical outcome: An APA task force report. Am J Psychiatry 142:155–162, 1985

Cowdry RW, Goodwin FK: Biological physiological predictors of drug response, in Handbook of Biological Psychiatry (Pt VI). Edited by van Praag HM, Lader MH, Rafaelsen OJ, et al. New York, Dekker, 1981

Cowdry RW, Wehr TA, Zis AP, et al: Thyroid abnormalities associated with rapid-cycling bipolar illness. Arch Gen Psychiatry 40:414–420, 1983

De Montigny C, Grunberg F, Mayer A, et al: Lithium induces rapid relief of depression in tricyclic antidepressant non-responders. Br J Psychiatry 138:252–256, 1981

Dunner DL, Patrick V, Fieve RR: Rapid-cycling manic-depressive patients. Compr Psychiatry 18:561–566, 1977

Feighner JP, Merideth CH, Warren CS, et al: A double-blind study of bupropion and placebo in depression. Am J Psychiatry 141:525–529, 1984

Gardner DL, Cowdry RW: Alprazolam-induced dyscontrol in borderline personality disorder. Am J Psychiatry 142:98–100, 1985

Gillin JC: The sleep therapies of depression. Prog Neuropsychopharmacol Biol Psychiatry 7:351–364, 1983

Gitlin M, Jamison KR: Lithium clinics: Theory and practice. Hosp Comm Psychiatry 35:363–368, 1984

Goodwin FK, Murphy DL, Bunney WE Jr: Lithium carbonate treatment in depression and mania: A longitudinal double-blind study. Arch Gen Psychiatry 21:486–496, 1969

Goodwin FK, Prange AJ Jr, Post RM, et al: Potentiation of antidepressant effects by L-triiodothyronine in tricyclic nonresponders. Am J Psychiatry 139:34–38, 1982

Heninger GR, Charney DS, Sternberg, DE: Lithium augmentation of antidepressant treatment: An effective prescription for treatment-refractory depression. Arch Gen Psychiatry 40:1335–1342, 1983

Jamison KR, Gerner RH, Goodwin FK: Patient and physician attitudes toward lithium: Relationship to compliance. Arch Gen Psychiatry 36:866–869, 1979

Kline NS, Cooper TB, Suckow RF, et al: Protection of patients on MAOIs against hypertensive crises. J Clin Psychopharmacol 1:410–411, 1981

Krauthammer C, Klerman GL: The epidemiology of mania, in Manic Illness. Edited by Shopsin B. New York, Raven Press, 1979

Oppenheim G: Estrogen in the treatment of depression: Neuropharmacological mechanisms. Biol Psychiatry 18:721–725, 1983

Pare CMB, Al-Mousawi M, Sandler M, et al: Attempts to attenuate the "cheese effect": Combined drug therapy in depressive illness. J Affective Disord 9:137–141, 1985

Post RM: Clinic perspective on the use of carbamazepine in manic–depressive illness. Fair Oaks Hospital Psychiatry Letter, 3, 1985

Post RM, Ballenger JC, Uhde TW, et al: Efficacy of carbamazepine in manic–depressive illness: Implications for underlying mechanisms, in

Neurobiology of Mood Disorders. Edited by Post RM, Ballenger JC. Baltimore, MD, Williams & Wilkins, 1984

Rosenthal NE, Sack DA, Carpenter CJ, et al: Antidepressant effects of light in seasonal affective disorder. Am J Psychiatry 142:163–170, 1985

Rudorfer MV, Golden RN, Potter WZ: Second generation antidepressants. Psychiatr Clin North Am 7:519–534, 1984

Sack DA, Nurnberger J, Rosenthal NE, et al: Potentiation of antidepressant medications by phase advance of the sleep-wake cycle. Am J Psychiatry 142:606–608, 1985

Schilgen B, Tolle R: Partial sleep deprivation as therapy for depression. Arch Gen Psychiatry 37:267–271, 1980

Schou M: Lithium as a prophylactic agent in unipolar affective illness. Arch Gen Psychiatry 36:849–851, 1979

Stancer HC, Persad E: Treatment of intractable rapid cycling manic–depressive disorder with levothyroxine: Clinical observations. Arch Gen Psychiatry 39:311–312, 1982

Wehr TA, Goodwin FK: Rapid cycling in manic–depressives induced by tricyclic antidepressants. Arch Gen Psychiatry 36:555–559, 1979

Wehr TA, Wirz-Justice A, Goodwin FK, et al: Phase advance of the circadian sleep–wake cycle as an antidepressant. Science 206:710–713, 1979

White KL, Simpson G: Combined MAOI tricyclic antidepressant treatment: A re-evaluation. J Clin Psychopharmacol 1:264–282, 1981

2

Pharmacological Treatment of Anxiety Disorders

Robert H. Gerner, M.D.

2

Pharmacological Treatment of Anxiety Disorders

DIAGNOSTIC CONSIDERATIONS

The specification of subgroups of anxiety disorders with implications for distinct pharmacological interventions was a recent development and is a major contribution of the *Diagnostic and Statistical Manual of Mental Disorders (Third Edition)* (*DSM-III;* American Psychiatric Association 1980). Because research to determine the most efficacious treatment is a function of these diagnoses, it is essential to evaluate carefully each patient by using the *DSM-III*. Anxiety disorders are broadly classified into phobic disorders and anxiety states. The Epidemiology Catchment Area study of the National Institute of Mental Health (NIMH) (Robins et al. 1984) has found that the prevalence of significant anxiety in our population is high: anxiety/somatization, 10–15 percent; phobias, 8–23 percent; obsessive–compulsive disorder, 2–3 percent; panic, 1.4 percent.

The essential feature of the phobic disorders is an irrational fear of a situation, an activity, or a specific object. Invariably the patient recognizes that the fear is excessive. When such fears are a source

The opinions presented in this chapter do not necessarily reflect the official position of the Veterans Administration.

of social dysfunction or enduring distress to the individual, the designation of a disorder can be made. There are three subtypes of phobic disorders: simple phobias, social phobias, and agoraphobia with or without panic attacks. Simple phobias are most common and are typically specific for an object (such as a cat) or a setting (as in acrophobia or claustrophobia). Only when exposed to that setting (or when thinking of it) does the individual become overwhelmingly fearful, often having symptoms similar to a panic attack (see below). However, anticipatory anxiety about the possibility of experiencing the phobic object can produce discomfort at other times. It is generally believed that most afflicted individuals live their lives "around their phobia" and do not seek treatment unless they cannot avoid the phobic object. Simple phobias that persist in adulthood generally do not spontaneously remit. Social phobias encompass those experiences commonly perceived as "stage fright." Situations that may expose one to scrutiny, humiliation, or embarrassment are avoided to an irrational extent, although the individual knows these avoidances are excessive. Typically, concern that others will detect the anxiety and fear enhances the phobic avoidance, setting up a vicious cycle. Specific situations include fear of speaking or performing in public, being called on in school, eating in public, or carrying out any ordinarily mundane activity (such as writing) in front of others. This disorder is considered rare and is often associated with generalized anxiety. One of its most disabling aspects is its interference with opportunities for social activities and job advancement.

Agoraphobia is a marked fear of being alone or of being in public places from which escape would be difficult or help unavailable. Thus crowds, streets, stores, freeways, tunnels, bridges, elevators, and so on provoke anxiety. Agoraphobic individuals often become quite dependent on others for constant reassurance. Agoraphobia may develop independently, but it more commonly occurs as a secondary symptom of panic attacks. It is hypothesized that in such cases the individual develops anticipatory anxiety of having a panic attack in one situation and then another. This is repeated over many months or years, and slowly restricts the individual's range of experience. The severity of agoraphobia

waxes and wanes over the years, sometimes with complete remission between episodes. The diagnosis is always specified as being
with or without panic attacks. Agoraphobic phenomena can occur
as a secondary feature of depression or social phobia and should be
so identified when appropriate.

Anxiety states are subgrouped into panic disorder, generalized
anxiety disorder, obsessive–compulsive disorder, and posttraumatic stress disorder. Panic disorder is unique in having sudden
onsets ("out of the blue") of an intense feeling of apprehension,
fear, terror, a sense of impending doom and dissolution, and often
a fear of "going crazy" or losing control. This state usually is
experienced subjectively as lasting for a timeless period, but typically lasts only a few minutes. Accompanying or immediately
after this subjective state are physiological signs and symptoms of
dyspnea, palpitations, chest discomfort, smothering, dizziness, ver-
tigo, depersonalization or derealization, paresthesias, diaphoresis,
tremors, agitation, and so forth. The onset of these attacks is
apparently random and usually begins in early adulthood. They
may come in clusters over weeks or months, then abate, only to
return in several months or years. A common course is for the
individual to rush for medical evaluation only to be told nothing
is wrong. This may be repeated several times, until the frustrated
patient no longer seeks help and adopts a more reclusive lifestyle.
Patients also attribute situational causality to each attack, and
subsequently avoid those settings involved (that is, restaurants,
grocery stores, parties, and so on). This may simulate agoraphobia
or social phobia, but really is conditioned avoidance. Not surpris-
ingly, anticipatory anxiety is also a complication of this disorder.
A genetic association of panic disorder with affective disorders has
been hypothesized, but remains controversial at this time.

Generalized anxiety disorder is characterized by enduring anxiety of greater than one month with signs of three of the following:
motor tension, autonomic hyperactivity, apprehensive expectation, or vigilance and scanning (feeling "on edge," impatient,
distractible, concentrating poorly, or having insomnia). Whereas
mild depression is commonly associated with this complex of
symptoms, care should be taken not to underdiagnose a depressive

episode that warrants treatment with antidepressants.

Obsessive–compulsive disorder is rare, with the essential features of recurrent obsessions (persistent ideas, thoughts, or impulses that are ego dystonic) and compulsions (repetitive and stereotyped behaviors). As with phobias, the individual usually recognizes the senselessness of these behaviors and finds them to be ego dystonic. Depression is a common concomitant feature, and should be considered as a primary diagnosis.

Posttraumatic stress disorder acute (less than six months' duration) and chronic or delayed (greater than six months' duration) can be identified when an event that is a stressor to almost everyone occurs prior to the development of symptoms of experiencing recurrent memories, dreams, or actual events of the traumatic incident. This is associated with a decrease in cathexsis to others, significant activities, or to one's own affect, as well as with two of the following: hyperalertness or startle response, sleep disturbance, guilt about surviving, difficulty concentrating, avoidance of remembering the event, and worsening of symptoms when the event is recalled by associating symbolic or similar events.

CLINICAL USE OF BENZODIAZEPINE ANXIOLYTICS

The treatment of anxiety and insomnia results in the greatest number of prescriptions for a class of medication in the world. Historically the sources for such medicines have ranged from opium in laudanum to alcoholic medicine-show remedies. Despite the widespread use of these agents, physicians are divided in opinion as to whether they are overprescribed (Heiman and Wood 1981). To some extent, the controversy over their use may partly be due to considering them in an oversimplified context. The traditional concept that anxiety is a symptom of a pure psychological conflict is giving way to newer concepts based on human and primate studies of endogenous anxiety syndromes (Sheehan et al. 1984; Skolnick and Paul 1983), of genetic relationships of some anxiety disorders to affective disorders, and to the discovery of endogenous benzodiazepine receptors in the brain (Hoehn-Saric 1982; Insel et al. 1984; Tallman et al. 1980). As we consider the

Table 1.   Anxiolytic/Hypnotic Agents

Agent
Benzodiazepines
Nonbenzodiazepines
buspirone
Barbiturates
Nonbarbiturate sedatives
chloral hydrate
ethchlorvynol
glutethimide
meprobamate
methyprylon
Other
β-receptor blockers
neuroleptics
antidepressants (tricyclic-like agents and monoamine oxidase inhibitors)
hydroxyzine and other antihistamines

vast number of current medications available for the generic conditions of anxiety/insomnia, it is convenient to organize medical
interventions into several clusters (Table 1). Each of these generic
groups has been used to treat one or more of the anxiety syndromes.

Major advances in the nomenclature and diagnostic reliability
of psychiatry have extended the number of disorders or symptom
complexes for which the anxiolytic agents may be appropriate,
either as the main treatment or as a treatment synergistic with
other medical, dynamic, cognitive, or behavioral therapies (Table
2). Because of the widespread use of benzodiazepine anxiolytics in
psychiatric practice, a major section of this chapter is devoted to
their use in clinical settings. Contrary to traditional lore and even
recent reviews, there are differences in efficacy and indications for
clinical use within the benzodiazepines and certainly among
benzodiazepines and other agents sharing similar indications. Any
consideration of this group of agents must bear on their potential
side effects as well as specific clinical issues affecting the choice
and/or dosing of the agent in particular clinical situations. These
factors include those listed in Table 3, and are discussed next.

Table 2.   Syndromes Responding to Anxiolytic Agents

Syndrome
Generalized anxiety disorder[a]
Panic disorder
Posttraumatic stress disorder
Phobias
Simple
Social
Agoraphobia
Withdrawal from alcohol and sedatives/hypnotics
Insomnia
Aggressive syndromes[b]
Depression
Manic and schizophrenic psychoses
Tardive dyskinesia

[a]This and the following five disorders/syndromes are indications for anxiolytic use.
[b]Anxiolytics may be useful for this and the following three disorders/syndromes.

Table 3.   Clinical Considerations for Anxiolytic Choice

Consideration
Dependence
Drug-diagnosis specificity
Drug interactions
Interaction with other organ systems
Lethality in overdose
Pseudodementia/memory impairment
Withdrawal potential

Note. Table 4 lists other characteristics of each drug that ought to be considered relevant to clinical decisions.

Specific indications for the benzodiazepine group of compounds include simple insomnia, generalized anxiety disorder, phobic disorders, panic disorder, agoraphobia with panic attacks, phobic avoidance, and to a lesser extent obsessive–compulsive disorder. Use of antidepressant drugs for anxiety disorders is discussed later in this chapter. The duration of symptom involvement that warrants medical intervention is not known. Specifically, this means it is not known what the spontaneous remission rate is during the early phases of anxiety disorders. If symptoms continue for four weeks and through the evaluation period, it seems reasonable to consider using medication. These agents have few differences in their mechanism of therapeutic activity at either the clinical or molecular level. Alprazolam and buspirone are mainly used as anxiolytics, triazolam as a hypnotic, and clonazepam as an anti-convulsant/antipsychotic sedative (Chouinard et al. 1983). Although the other benzodiazepines are often suggested as indicated for either anxiety or insomnia, there is little scientific evidence to support such a discrimination, with the possible exception of alprazolam for use with panic disorders. Although several studies show that alprazolam is more efficacious than other benzodiazepines for panic disorders with or without agoraphobia (Sheehan 1982; Sheehan et al. 1984), additional studies from several other centers are needed to document these findings with certainty.

Prior to starting anxiolytics/hypnotics the clinician should document that the patient has been informed of potential sedation, risks of driving or operating heavy machinery, and of synergistic sedative effects when combined with other drugs or alcohol. It may be wise to inform the patient that abrupt discontinuation may produce serious withdrawal symptoms and that conception should be avoided. Table 4 shows common initial and daily oral dose ranges for adults. Adolescents and geriatric patients may tolerate only lower doses. Because of the wide interindividual range of metabolism, one should also consider that a significant number of patients will need large doses to achieve anxiolytic effects, and that such patients are not necessarily abusing the medication (Laughren et al. 1982).

It is easier to determine when to initiate treatment than when to terminate it. Most patients have been shown to use benzodiazepines irregularly depending on the occurrence of potentially stressful situations (Mellinger et al. 1985). A short-term course of treatment for anxiety (six weeks) has been shown to be adequate for approximately 50 percent of patients over a four-month follow-up (Rickels et al. 1983b, 1984). However, over 12 months of follow-up more than 50 percent reexperience symptoms, and they are severe in 30 percent. Thus a significant number

Table 4. Oral Dosages of Anxiolytics

Drug	Trade Name	Common Dosage range/day (mg)[a]	Half-life[b]
Alprazolam	Xanax	0.25–6	Short
Buspirone	BuSpar	5–50	Short
Chlorazepate	Tranxene	7.5–60	Long
Chlordiazepoxide	Librium	10–100	Long
Clonazepam	Clonopin	0.25–4	Intermediate
Diazepam	Valium	2–50	Long
Flurazepam	Dalmane	15–30	Long
Halazepam	Paxipam	20–160	Long
Lorazepam	Ativan	1–8	Short
Oxazepam	Serax	10–100	Intermediate
Prazepam	Centrax	10–60	Long
Temazepam	Restoril	10–60	Intermediate
Triazolam	Halcion	0.25–1	Ultrashort

[a]Common clinical dosage is typically in the middle of the range shown. Short and intermediate half-life compounds are usually given in divided doses, with a frequency of at least one dose per half-life.
[b]Half-life as shown is generalized. Table 5 gives more specific information.

of patients may benefit from prolonged treatment. Panic disorders are recurrent and continued treatment with either a constant or intermittent pattern is the norm. Fears that anxiolytic use might lead to an ever-increasing number of drug-dependent adults do not appear to be substantiated (Mellinger et al. 1984). Patients did not take ever-increasing doses of benzodiazepines; instead they were found to use them judiciously. This may be contrasted to the barbiturates and similar drugs where tolerance develops quickly, and patients commonly increase the dose incrementally over time. The difference may be that patients do not seem to develop tolerance to the anxiolytic effects of benzodiazepines and are therefore willing to stay at a therapeutic dose.

Depression and Benzodiazepines

The differential diagnosis of depression and anxiety is relatively straightforward in some situations, but in clinical practice there is frequently evidence for both disorders, and treatment often must be initiated while the evaluation continues. The issue of anxiolytic/hypnotic use in depressed patients is twofold: a) concomitant use with bona fide antidepressants and b) their use as a specific antidepressant agent. By the late 1970s there was a consensus that the available evidence did not support specific antidepressant qualities of the benzodiazepines (Shatzberg and Cole 1978). Of the approximately 20 studies reported by that time that used double-blind methods and comparison to an antidepressant, benzodiazepines were inferior in half and more or less equivalent in half. However, many of these patients might not meet our current *DSM-III* diagnoses of major affective or primary affective disorder, and may more appropriately have been mild or mixed anxious/ depressives. An interest in potential antidepressant effects of these compounds continues because of their relative safety compared with the tricyclic antidepressants and monoamine oxidase inhibitors (MAOIs). Recent investigations with relatively large doses of alprazolam (up to 4.5 mg/day) in double-blind, placebo-controlled trials for major depression have supported the hypothesis that it was equally efficacious as imipramine (up to 225 mg/day), and had fewer side effects other than sedation (Feighner et al. 1983). Although this was a large multicenter study with 723 patients, its results need replication. Presently, standard antidepressants are relatively more indicated for the initial treatment of uncomplicated depression. The adjuvant use anxiolytics/hypnotics during antidepressant treatment appears to be best decided based on clinical judgment and observation of patient response. There are no specific contraindications to their use. However, fixed-dose combination benzodiazepine/tricyclic antidepressants do not conform to the clinical need to adjust medication treatment to alterations in a patient's behavioral status.

Pharmacokinetic Considerations in Using Benzodiazepines

The major bases for clinical choice rest on the differences in half-life and the mode of metabolism (Table 5). For individuals with chronic anxiety throughout the day, treatment with a long

Table 5. Metabolism of Common Anxiolytics

Drug	Half-life (hours)	Metabolic Mechanism	Active Metabolite
Chlordiazepoxide	30	Oxidative	Desmethyldiazepam and others
Diazepam	25–60	Oxidative	Desmethyldiazepam (T ½ = 30–200; desmethyldiazepam is metabolized to oxazepam[a])
Chlorazepate	30–60	Oxidative	
Prazepam	30–60	Oxidative	
Halazepam	30–60	Oxidative	
Flurazepam	30–60	Oxidative	Desalkylflurazepam (T ½ = 100)
Temazepam	10–20	Glucuronidation	
Lorazepam	10–20	Glucuronidation	None
Alprazolam	6–20	Oxidative	
Oxazepam	5–15	Glucuronidation	
Triazolam	1–4	Oxidative	None
Clonazepam	18–50	Oxidative	
Buspirone	2–9	Oxidative	1–2-Pyrimidinyl–piperazine

[a]This active metabolite is the same for chlorazepate, prazepam, and halazepam.

half-life compound gives a continuous blood level of anxiolytic. Patients on short half-life benzodiazepines often report that they can "feel" the drug wearing off after four to six hours. This warrants attention because such reports correspond to a phase of decreasing blood levels. Similarly, for insomnia that occurs beyond the middle of the night (and after a diagnosis of depression and appropriate antidepressants have been considered), the longer acting benzodiazepines offer continued hypnotic effect. Patients with difficulty falling asleep or acute situational anxiety may benefit more from short-acting agents. Long-acting agents may be overly sedative once the anxious situation has passed. In these acute situations it is also important to realize that the anxiolytics are of more use in preventing the initiation and development of anxiety than in reversing anxiety syndromes. Thus, if a junior executive consistently has severe anxiety during board meetings, he or she should take a short-acting agent one-half to one hour before the meeting rather than a long-acting agent after anxiety has become moderate or severe. A short-acting agent will not produce lethargy after the acute anxiety-provoking situation is resolved. Such medical management appropriately opens the door, of course, to combining behavioral and pharmacological treatments (Muskin and Fyer 1981; Taylor et al. 1982). Thus, benzodiazepines may enhance treatment with systematic desensitization.

Another important aspect of half-life is that it takes approximately four to five half-lives to reach a steady state. However, the drug must be given at least as often as the half-life to achieve a steady state (Greenblatt et al. 1984). Thus, patients who take short-acting benzodiazepines and who have chronic anxiety may experience recurrent symptoms during the day as the drug wears off, or may possibly even develop some withdrawal symptoms. If anxiolytic treatment is chronic, it may be advisable to select longer acting agents or to direct the patient to take the drug several times throughout the day. Because benzodiazepine half-lives vary considerably between individuals (especially with the oxidatively metabolized group), it is not uncommon to find patients who do not rapidly metabolize the drug developing very high levels of the longer acting benzodiazepines. Such patients may appear confused as well as sedated and it is therefore important not to increase their anxiolytic to treat agitation resulting from iatrogenically induced confusion. This is particularly important for longer half-life drugs in the older population (Salzman et al. 1983) and in individuals with liver impairment.

Although it is true that the very lowest plasma levels cannot be expected to have a clinical effect, a true correlation of efficacy or side effects to a threshold blood level or to the concept of a therapeutic window has not consistently been demonstrated with benzodiazepines. The few studies to date have been with diazepam or chlordiazepoxide. Some significant findings have been reported, but the clinician must be aware that plasma level measurements vary substantially between laboratories, and it is not even clear which parent/metabolite is the most useful to measure. For example, many of the benzodiazepines have active metabolites, and for some the parent compound is relatively inactive.

Table 6. Parenteral Benzodiazepine Dosage

Drug	Intramuscular Dosage (mg)[a]	Intravenous Dosage (mg)
Chlordiazepoxide	50 (25–100)	Rarely used
Diazepam	5 (2–20)	5–10 (slowly, at least 1 min/5 mg)
Lorazepam	2 (2–4)	2 (slowly)

[a]Common clinical mean and range are shown.

However, blood level determinations are useful when toxicity is suspected. A positive correlation of diazepam plasma levels with response has been reported, with therapeutic responses tending to occur to a greater extent when levels were greater than 300–400 ng/ml (Bowden and Fisher 1982; Dasberg et al. 1974, respectively). Two of the metabolites of chlordiazepoxide, desmethylchlordiazepoxide and demoxepam, reportedly are positively correlated with anxiety reduction, but "therapeutic levels" have not been substantiated (Lin and Friedel 1979).

Three benzodiazepines are available for parenteral use: diazepam, chlordiazepoxide, and lorazepam (Table 6). Although all three can be used intravenously, diazepam and lorazepam are usually selected for intravenous use to achieve sedation, for medical procedures, and to break an epileptic seizure. Diazepam and chlordiazepoxide are unpredictably absorbed after intramuscular injection and are therefore relatively less useful by this route in most clinical settings. Lorazepam, in contrast, is rapidly absorbed and produces less pain because it does not precipitate at physiological pH. However, all benzodiazepines can produce painful sterile abscesses if perivascular extravasation occurs. Lorazepam and diazepam both relieve acute anxiety within one hour (approximately 3 mg and 10 mg/60 kg, respectively). When given intravenously, diazepam is more rapidly distributed and metabolized than lorazepam. Thus lorazepam has a more prolonged clinical effect, often producing an anterograde amnesia for several hours longer than diazepam. Apnea is a not uncommon complication of intravenous diazepam treatment, and patients who receive it should be supervised by medical personnel who can maintain artificial respiration. Clinical reports suggest that lorazepam may have a lower apneic potential. Slow infusion is the best means of preventing apnea.

Drug-Drug Interactions Involving Benzodiazepines

There are few major interactions of benzodiazepines with other drugs. They are additive to some extent in producing sedation when combined with other sedative agents, but it is not a common clinical problem with antidepressants. However, there is clear evidence that neuropsychological test performance is diminished when alcohol and benzodiazepines are combined (Lister and File 1983; Palva et al. 1979). Regrettably, such studies have not shown whether this is to a greater extent than would be observed with the additional ingestion of alcohol or benzodiazepine alone. In contrast to the benzodiazepines, buspirone does not enhance the psychomotor effects of alcohol either with acute or chronic buspirone use (Moskowitz and Smiley 1982).

There are two major metabolic pathways for the common anxiolytics. Most are metabolized by oxidation in the liver, whereas a few are conjugated through glucuronidation and excreted in the urine. There are virtually no clinically significant physiological effects on the latter metabolic pathway, but numerous drugs and hepatic conditions can alter the oxidative metabolism of many of these compounds and produce clinically significant effects for patients receiving them.

Table 7 shows the effects of various parameters on benzodiazepine metabolism. These effects are only clinically important when ancillary drugs or disease states change during benzodiazepine treatment. Occasionally such alterations may explain toxicity or inefficacy. Chronic alcohol use induces hepatic oxidative metabolism and may therefore increase the metabolism of some benzodiazepines. Disulfiram (Antabuse) decreases hepatic oxidative metabolism and therefore substantially increases the half-life of some benzodiazepines. Propranolol also inhibits oxidative metabolism and increases oxidatively metabolized benzo-

Table 7. Effect of Drugs and Other Factors on Metabolically Oxidized Anxiolytics

Increases anxiolytic level
  Disulfiram
  Estrogens (oral contraceptives)
  Cimetidine
  Propranolol
  Isoniazide
  Propoxyphene
  Age
  Hepatic disease
Decreases anxiolytic level
  Alcohol
  Coffee
  Tobacco smoking

diazepines' half-life, although the clinical significance of this is debatable. Oral contraceptives impair clearance and thus increase the half-life of hepatically oxidized benzodiazepines. The widely prescribed antiulcer agent cimetidine interferes with the hepatic metabolism of diazepam and probably other hepatically oxidized benzodiazepines shown in Table 5. Thus, higher blood levels may occur with ordinary doses. However, the evidence does not suggest that this is of much clinical significance (Greenblatt et al. 1984). Both coffee and the tar in tobacco smoke stimulate the synthesis of hepatic enzymes that may result in decreased drug levels (Downing and Rickels 1981). This finding is of little consequence unless coffee consumption and smoking habits are changed. The main clinical consequences relevant to drug–drug interactions occur if these drugs are either instituted or discontinued during anxiolytic treatment. Even then there is rarely a robust clinical change except in the aged or individuals with hepatic disease.

Side Effects of Benzodiazepines

Benzodiazepines have few effects on organs other than the brain. Diazepam and chlordiazepoxide increase coronary blood flow and cardiac output and decrease heart rate and systolic blood pressure in dogs but probably do not have clinically significant direct cardiovascular effects at normal doses in humans. Further, they do not induce hepatic enzyme synthesis as do the barbiturates. On the other hand, the benzodiazepines interact significantly with liver function. Decreased liver function associated with aging or liver disease markedly decreases the breakdown of benzodiazepines metabolized by oxidative enzymes. Thus, the half-life of drugs such as diazepam or chlordiazepoxide may increase sixfold, resulting in clinically significant high blood levels from ordinary doses given to aged or hepatically ill patients (Shader and Greenblatt 1982). Such high blood levels may produce a pseudodementia syndrome or aggravate preexisting confusion. This metabolic effect does not appear to occur with benzodiazepines that are metabolized by glucuronidation.

The major side effect of benzodiazepines is central nervous system depression resulting in drowsiness and impairment of intellectual functioning. This depression has nothing to do with the mood or illness of depression, however. As discussed previously, there is some evidence for an antidepressant effect of benzodiazepines in some studies. Worsening of mental depression has been reported rarely with the administration of relatively large doses of diazepam in some patients with mixed anxiety/depression (Hall and Joffe 1972) or endogenous major depression (Bowen 1978). These are isolated findings and must be taken in the context of the many studies showing either no effect or a mild antidepressant effect of benzodiazepines (see for example Shatzberg and Cole 1978). Most individuals develop a tolerance to daytime drowsiness when taking stable daily doses of benzodiazepines within a few days of reaching steady-state plasma levels. Continued drowsiness is an indication to reevaluate the dosage and need for anxiolytics. Buspirone (a nonbenzodiazepine) and to a lesser extent alprazolam (Aden and Thein 1980; Rickels et al. 1983a) and prazepam (Shader et al. 1984) appear to be less sedating than the traditional benzodiazepines. A "hangover" effect after hypnotic use has been related to the long half-life of some of the benzodiazepines (see Table 6). Switching to a shorter acting agent generally reduces this effect.

Memory impairment and pseudodementia may occur with all of the benzodiazepines when measured on sophisticated neuropsychological tests. However, except as a secondary effect to sedation, significant impairments of common tasks of daily living and working have not been consistently shown. Typically, memory effects are acute and dose dependent (Linnoila et al. 1983) and are especially evident with parenteral use. This is the basis for using intravenous diazepam or lorazepam as amnesics for unpleasant medical procedures. The memory impairment itself appears to be a defect in consolidation. Thus, patients can cooperate and follow directions, but are subsequently amnesic. Some investigators have suggested that the impairment is secondary to sleepiness (Roth et al. 1980). Others, however, have suggested that impairment with usual oral doses is more specifically associated with the short-acting agents (Sharf et al. 1984) and/or during the initial phases of benzodiazepine treatment. It is important to note that the long-term use of benzodiazepines at normal clinical doses does not seem to affect psychomotor performance (Lucki et al. 1985). However, if memory is affected, it may be specific to the benzodiazepines, as it has not been found to happen with narcotics compared with benzodiazepines (Hendler et al. 1980), nor with buspirone. The older barbiturates and similar compounds have been studied with less interest, but are generally considered to produce some decrements in memory function.

Disinhibition of behavior is a euphemism suggesting a pathophysiology for hostile, aggressive, or irritable behavior occurring with minimal provocation in patients on sedatives/hypnotics. This effect may occur with alcohol, barbiturates, and benzodiazepines and has been reported in normals as well as identified patients. The benzodiazepines most commonly associated with this phenomenon are diazepam and chlordiazepoxide, although the incidence in clinical settings is unknown. Few other agents have been specifically evaluated for this effect, but oxazepam, in comparison with the two agents just mentioned, reportedly does not produce such effects. The barbiturate-like agents also can produce such disinhibition syndromes.

Death from overdose is often associated with ingestion of

anxiolytic drugs. Because patients appear to overdose using medication at their disposal (Busto et al. 1980), common sense suggests using less lethal compounds. This is particularly true because the prediction of suicide is totally unreliable (Murphy 1983; Pokorny 1983), and because patients often keep medication for years, over which time their mental status may change. Overdoses with benzodiazepines require fewer medical hospitalizations and cause fewer disturbances of consciousness than other older types of sedatives/hypnotics. The most lethal compounds in this group are the barbiturates, nonbarbiturates, and chloral hydrate. The least lethal are buspirone (which does not appear to depress respiratory or cardiovascular activity) and the benzodiazepines. Because death occurs extremely rarely from any benzodiazepine-only overdose, we cannot predict a lethality index across the various benzodiazepines.

Cholestatic jaundice has been rarely reported in association with diazepam, chlordiazepoxide, and flurazepam. The mechanism for this is unknown, as is its cross-sensitivity with other benzodiazepines. Cerebral atrophy had been suggested as a sequela of benzodiazepine abuse, but more thorough studies have documented that benzodiazepine abusers have computed tomography (CT) scans that are similar to normal controls. Atrophic changes are apparently related to alcohol abuse by these patients, independent of benzodiazepines (Poser et al. 1983). Teratogenicity has been reported after their use in the first trimester, possibly causing cleft lip. Further, animal studies have shown behavioral effects in offspring after benzodiazepines were given to the mother during the last trimester (Kellogg et al. 1980). This area is still controversial both for diazepam as well as all other sedatives/hypnotics/anxiolytics. Current practice and forensic considerations should caution against prescribing any such medication during pregnancy.

Because benzodiazepines have anticonvulsant activity, it should not be surprising that some effect on electroconvulsive therapy (ECT) was found. Benzodiazepines given during the period of ECT treatment either as a hypnotic or for daytime sedation reportedly significantly reduce the duration of seizures, were associated with more "missed" seizures, and resulted in more treatments (Stromgren et al. 1980). This suggests that the use of other agents such as buspirone, chloral hydrate, or hydroxyzine is relatively more indicated.

Benzodiazepine Withdrawal Phenomena

Until recently, clinically significant withdrawal was thought to be quite rare unless benzodiazepines were used at high doses for a prolonged period of time. By 1977 fewer than 50 cases had been reported (Herxheimer 1977). The current incidence of withdrawal symptoms varies greatly between surveys, but commonly ranges around 25 percent of patients who have taken benzodiazepines for several months (Hallstrom and Lader 1981). That such a phenomenon is due to the benzodiazepine and not to the patient's underlying anxiety is supported by the lack of withdrawal symptoms in placebo-treated comparison groups. Withdrawal syndromes depend on drug half-life, with short half-life agents having an earlier onset and possibly a greater liability for withdrawal than longer half-life agents (Fontaine et al. 1985). Thus, early morning insomnia as a sign of benzodiazepine withdrawal may occur during daily treatment with ultrashort-acting agents (Kales et al. 1983), whereas seizures after abrupt withdrawal from long-acting agents may not occur for two weeks. Withdrawal symptoms may also be affected by the inherent anxiolytic, hypnotic, anticonvulsant, and possibly antipsychotic activity of the benzodiazepines.

Initial withdrawal symptoms typically resemble the anxiety symptoms for which treatment was initiated, thus making it difficult to differentiate relapse from withdrawal. Reviewing the reported cases shows that interindividual differences are very large and that careful consideration should be given to the occurrence of a withdrawal phenomenon before concluding the patient is manipulating, having an hysterical conversion, or any other dynamic interpretation. Withdrawal symptoms are relatively more likely with the short half-life agents than with others. Table 8 lists the range of these withdrawal symptoms.

Patients undergoing withdrawal typically evidence several of

Table 8. Symptoms of Benzodiazepine Withdrawal

Symptom	
Akathesia-like restlessness	Tremulousness
Increased energy/hypomania	Diaphoresis and tachycardia
Impaired concentration	Hypersensitivity to light and/or sound
Organic brain syndrome (reversible)	Initial, middle, and terminal insomnia
Emotional irritability (often preceding convulsion)	Gastrointestional symptoms
	Anorexia
Neuromuscular irritability	Nausea
Agitation	Vomiting
Depersonalization	Cramps
Depression	Fear/apprehension
Headache	Myoclonus
Paresthesias, hypesthesias	Ataxia
Anxiety	Acute psychosis
	Grand mal convulsions

these symptoms. Prediction of withdrawal for an individual is quite imprecise. Severe withdrawal has been reported after long exposure (months) to low doses, but has also occurred after only several weeks of taking "normal" doses. Certainly anyone taking benzodiazepines for several months (even at low doses) may be expected to show some withdrawal if they are abruptly discontinued (Winokur et al. 1980). A substantial amount of investigative data demonstrates that tapering doses by one-third every week will prevent withdrawal for both short- and long-acting benzodiazepines (Chouinard et al. 1983) if the duration of treatment has been a matter of weeks. However, after long-term treatment, even gradual tapering may produce significant withdrawal (Petursson and Lader 1981). The duration of the withdrawal may last from four to six weeks and longer (up to four months) in chronic users. Retreatment with benzodiazepines immediately relieves the symptoms and allows the clinician to taper the patient more gradually. It is especially useful when discontinuing short-acting agents to temporarily change the patient to a long-acting benzodiazepine because the longer acting drug has a slower rate of decrease in blood levels as it is withdrawn. This strategy is also appropriate when changing from other anxiolytics to the nonbenzodiazepine buspirone, which does not show cross-tolerance with the benzodiazepines/barbiturates, and does not prevent their withdrawal syndrome. Patients who show neuromuscular and emotional irritability probably should be restarted on benzodiazepines at adequate doses to reduce these symptoms, as this symptom constellation indicates brain irritability and increased vulnerability to a seizure. Tyrer and Owen (1983) report that patients with personality characteristics of lability, resourcelessness, sensitivity, and impulsiveness may be more likely to experience withdrawal.

USE OF ANTIDEPRESSANT DRUGS FOR ANXIETY DISORDERS

Both the tricyclic-like antidepressants and MAOIs clearly demonstrate robust therapeutic effects in the treatment of some types of anxiety disorders. Clinical experience and initial studies (Sheehan 1982) suggest that both panic attacks and agoraphobia with panic attacks as well as posttraumatic stress syndrome respond somewhat better to MAOIs than tricyclic-like agents. Further, with the exception of alprazolam, these agents are more effective than the benzodiazepines. However, the nature of the patient's symptoms may make a consideration of the risks with the MAOI agents difficult for patients to accept. Combined treatment with antidepressants and behavior therapy acts synergistically to greatly enhance the recovery rate compared with behavior therapy alone (from 20 to 60 or 90 percent) (DuPont 1982; Sheehan 1982). Therapeutic dosages have generally been found to parallel those for antidepressant use, although a significant minority respond to very low doses of tricyclic-like agents (25 mg imipramine equivalents). Because of this possibility and because anxious patients may be especially concerned about side effects, it is best to start with low doses and increase them gradually.

Obsessive–compulsive disorder has not been shown to respond well to benzodiazepines alone, and their use seems limited mainly to reducing secondary anxiety. Many isolated cases report that tricyclic-like antidepressants and MAOIs are occasionally effective. The tricyclic clomipramine (Anafranil) is considered an effective treatment and is the standard initial treatment in Europe and Great Britain. Regrettably, it is not available in the United States.

OTHER AGENTS FOR ANXIETY SYNDROMES

β-Adrenoceptor Blocking Agents

The systematic use of β-blockers for anxiety is relatively new. Most studies report that they are modestly effective for anxiety reduction but are less effective for psychic anxiety than benzodiazepines. Somatic anxiety manifested by tachycardia, tachipnea, tremors, and sweating respond equally well to β-blockers as to diazepam. The β-blockers are also effective for stage fright and possibly for other anticipation-anxiety situations (Peet 1984). However, they apparently are not effective for specific phobias (Bernadt et al. 1980), and their use for panic attacks is under continued evaluation. The combination of a β-blocker and a benzodiazepine has been reported to be synergistic and without additional side effects (Hallstrom et al. 1981). The β-blockers have an advantage of not producing dependence (in contrast with benzodiazepines), and so may be especially useful for patients susceptible to drug dependence.

The dosage of β-blockers has to be individualized, and evidence indicates that the dose should be sufficient to decrease the resting pulse by eight or more beats/min (Hallstrom et al. 1981). Patients should be instructed to take their pulse once daily and to hold their medication if the pulse is below 60 beats/min. Initial propranolol dosage in adults is 40 mg/day and may be increased every 3 to 7 days up to 240 mg/day. Higher doses may be used with consideration. Side effects may include insomnia, impotence, nausea, bradycardia, orthostatic hypotension, exacerbation of congestive heart failure, and precipitation of asthma (except for atenolol). Individuals with cardiovascular disease should be treated in collaboration with an internist. Virtually all studies have used propranolol, although it is likely that other drugs would also be effective if they act through peripheral mechanisms (an as yet unknown conjecture). Propranolol confers some risk for inducing depression in doses above 100 mg/day and this possibility may be decreased by using atenolol or practolol, which do not as readily cross the blood-brain barrier. Initial anxiolytic studies with such agents suggest they are effective (Bonn et al. 1972).

Neuroleptics

Agitation may be usefully contrasted with anxiety as indicative of separate treatment strategies. Agitation is commonly associated with a physiological sense of restlessness, particularly as a component of unipolar depression in some patients. Both clinical experience and studies have indicated that low doses of neuroleptics are quite effective for reducing such agitation. Few studies have carefully compared neuroleptics and anxiolytics in nonschizophrenic populations, so conclusions regarding their relative efficacy cannot be validly made. Because of the risk of tardive dyskinesia, the use of neuroleptics for anxiety per se is commonly reserved for patients who have not responded to anxiolytics.

Barbiturates and Nonbarbiturate Sedatives/Hypnotics

Although the barbiturates have been used in clinical practice for decades, their exact mode of molecular action has not been precisely defined. Their anxiolytic action may be similar to that of the benzodiazepines, which are linked to activity at γ-aminobutyric acid receptor sites. The barbiturates have no advantages over benzodiazepine anxiolytics/hypnotics except a predictable anesthesia. Their use is generally limited to clinical situations when acute sedation is required for clinical management. Their potential for addiction and their low lethal dose make outpatient use difficult to justify in psychiatric patients. Chloral hydrate is a short-acting (five to eight hours) sedative frequently used for inpatients. However, similar to barbiturates, it is addictive and withdrawal can be severe. It is potentiated by alcohol and can be lethal in overdose. Ethchlorvynol is a rapidly acting and short-duration hypnotic, whereas meprobamate, glutethimide, and methyprylon are longer acting agents. All have major addiction potential, severe withdrawal syndromes, and are lethal when several days' doses are ingested. Thus, except for rare instances, the use of both the barbiturate and nonbarbiturate sedatives/hypnotics should be discouraged, especially for outpatients.

Antihistamines such as hydroxyzine possess sedative activity rather than anxiolytic activity per se. Although they are useful for intermittent acute sedation, their inherent antihistaminic properties produce unpleasant side effects such as drying the mucosa and impairing psychomotor performance.

SUMMARY

In conclusion, recent investigations have demonstrated that antidepressant agents are effective for some of the anxiety syndromes and that the anxiolytics have a wider application than has been traditional. Anxiolytics are more effective in preventing the development or escalation of anxiety than in acutely reversing it. The sophisticated use of these agents requires an appreciation of their basic pharmacokinetics, with special attention paid to clinical half-life and factors that affect it.

REFERENCES

Aden GC, Thein SG: Alprazolam compared to diazepam and placebo in the treatment of anxiety. J Clin Psychiatry 41:245–248, 1980

Bernadt MW, Silverstone T, Singleton W: Behavioural and subjective effects of beta-adrenergic blockade in phobic subjects. Br J Psychiatry 137:452–457, 1980

Bonn JA, Turner P, Hicks DC: Beta-adrenergic blockade with practolol in treatment of anxiety. Lancet 1:814, 1972

Bowden CL, Fisher JG: Relationship of diazepam serum level to antianxiety effects. J Clin Psychopharmacol 2:110–114, 1982

Bowen, RC: The effect of diazepam on the recovery of endogenously depressed patients. J Clin Pharmacol 18:280–284, 1978

Busto U, Kaplan HL, Sellers EM: Benzodiazepine-associated emergencies in Toronto. Am J Psychiatry 137:225–227, 1980

Chouinard G, Young SN, Annable L: Antimanic effect of clonazepam. Biol Psychiatry 18:451–466, 1983

Dasberg JJ, van der Kleijn, Guelen PJP: Plasma concentrations of diazepam and of its metabolite n-desmethyldiazepam in relation to anxiolytic effect. Clin Pharmacol Ther 15:473–483, 1974

Downing RW, Rickels K: Coffee consumption, cigarette smoking and reporting of drowsiness in anxious patients treated with benzodiazepines or placebo. Acta Psychiatr Scand 64:398–408, 1981

DuPont RL: Profile of a phobia treatment program: two-year follow-up, in Phobia: A Comprehensive Summary of Modern Treatments. Edited by DuPont RL. New York, Brunner/Mazel, 1982

Feighner JP, Aden GC, Fabre LF, et al: Comparison of alprazolam, imipramine, and placebo in the treatment of depression. JAMA 249:3057–3064, 1983

Fontaine R, Annable L, Beaudry P, et al: Efficacy and withdrawal of two potent benzodiazepines: bromazepam and lorazepam. Psychopharmacol Bull 21:91–92, 1985

Greenblatt DJ, Abernethy DR, Morse DS, et al: Clinical importance of the interaction of diazepam and cimetidine. N Engl J Med 310:1639–1643, 1984

Hall RCW, Joffe JR: Aberrant response to diazepam: a new syndrome. Am J Psychiatry 129:738–742, 1972

Hallstrom C, Treasaden I, Edwards JG, et al: Diazepam, propranolol and their combination in the management of chronic anxiety. Br J Psychiatry 139:417–421, 1981

Hallstrom C, Lader M: Benzodiazepine withdrawal phenomena. International Journal of Pharmacopsychiatry 16:235–244, 1981

Heiman EM, Wood G: Patient characteristics and clinician attitudes influencing the prescribing of benzodiazepines. J Clin Psychiatry 42:71–73, 1981

Hendler N, Cimini C, Ma T, et al: A comparison of cognitive impairment due to benzodiazepines and to narcotics. Am J Psychiatry 137:828–830, 1980

Herxheimer A: Physical dependence on benzodiazepines. Drug Ther Bull 15:22–30, 1977

Hoehn-Saric R: Neurotransmitters in anxiety. Arch Gen Psychiatry 39:735–742, 1982

Insel TR, Ninan PT, Aloi J, et al: A benzodiazepine receptor-mediated model of anxiety. Arch Gen Psychiatry 41:741–750, 1984

Kales A, Soldatos CR, Bixler EO, et al: Early morning insomnia with rapidly eliminated benzodiazepines. Science 220:95–97, 1983

Kellogg C, Tervo D, Ison J, et al: Prenatal exposure to diazepam alters behavioral development in rats. Science 207:205–207, 1980

Laughren TP, Battey YW, Greenblatt DJ: Chronic diazepam treatment in psychiatric outpatients. J Clin Psychiatry 43:461–462, 1982

Lin KM, Friedel RO: Relationship of plasma levels of chlordiazepoxide and metabolites to clinical response. Am J Psychiatry 136:18–23, 1979

Linnoila M, Erwin CW, Brendle A, et al: Psychomotor effects of diazepam in anxious patients and healthy volunteers. J Clin Psychopharmacol 3:88–96, 1983

Lister RG, File SE: Performance impairment and increased anxiety resulting from the combination of alcohol and lorazepam. J Clin Psychopharmacol 3:66–71, 1983

Lucki I, Rickels K, Geller AM: Psychomotor performance following the long-term use of benzodiazepines. Psychopharmacol Bull 21:93–96, 1985

Mellinger GD, Balter MB, Uhlenhuth EH: Prevalence and correlates of the long-term regular use of anxiolytics. JAMA 251:375–379, 1984

Mellinger GD, Balter MB, Uhlenhuth EH: Insomnia and its treatment: prevalence and correlates. Arch Gen Psychiatry 42:225–232, 1985

Moskowitz H, Smiley A: Effects of chronically administered buspirone and diazepam on driving-related skills performance. J Clin Psychiatry 43:45–55, 1982

Murphy GE: On suicide prediction and prevention. Arch Gen Psychiatry 40:343–344, 1983

Muskin PR, Fyer AJ: Treatment of panic disorder. J Clin Psychopharmacol 1:81–90, 1981

Palva ES, Linnoila M, Saario I, et al: Acute and subacute effects of diazepam on psychomotor skills: interaction with alcohol. Acta Pharmacol Toxicol 45:257–264, 1979

Peet M: Beta-blockade in anxiety. Postgrad Med J 60 (Suppl. 2):16–18, 1984

Petursson H, Lader MH: Withdrawal from long-term benzodiazepine treatment. Br Med J 283:643–645, 1981

Pokorny A: Prediction of suicide in psychiatric patients. Arch Gen Psychiatry 40:249–257, 1983

Poser W, Poser S, Roscher D, et al: Do benzodiazepines cause cerebral atrophy? Lancet 1:715, 1983

Rickels K, Csanalosi I, Greisman P, et al: A controlled clinical trial of alprazolam for the treatment of anxiety. JAMA 140:82–85, 1983a

Rickels K, Case GW, Downing RW, et al: Long-term diazepam therapy and clinical outcome. JAMA 250:767–771, 1983b

Rickels K, Case GW, Winokur A, et al: Long-term benzodiazepine therapy: benefits and risks. Psychopharmacol Bull 20:608–615, 1984

Robins LN, Helzer JE, Weissman MM, et al: Lifetime prevalence of specific psychiatric disorder in three sites. Arch Gen Psychiatry 41:949–958, 1984

Roth T, Hartse KM, Saab PG, et al: The effects of flurazepam, lorazepam and triazolam on sleep and memory. Psychopharmacology 70:231–237, 1980

Salzman C, Shader RI, Greenblatt DJ, et al: Long vs. short half-life benzodiazepines in the elderly. Arch Gen Psychiatry 40:293–295, 1983

Shader RI, Greenblatt DJ: Management of anxiety in the elderly: the balance between therapeutic and adverse effects. J Clin Psychiatry 43:8–16, 1982

Shader RI, Pary RJ, Harmatz JS, et al: Plasma concentrations and clinical effects after single oral doses of prazepam, clorazepate, and diazepam. J Clin Psychiatry 45:411–413, 1984

Sharf MB, Khosla N, Brocker N, et al: Differential amnestic properties of short- and long-acting benzodiazepines. J Clin Psychiatry 45:51–53, 1984

Shatzberg AF, Cole JO: Benzodiazepines in depressive disorders. Arch Gen Psychiatry 35:1359–1365, 1978

Sheehan DV: Current perspectives in the treatment of panic and phobic disorders. Drug Ther 12:179–193, 1982

Sheehan DV, Bao BC, Coleman JH, et al: Some biochemical correlates of panic attacks with agoraphobia and their response to a new treatment. J Clin Psychopharmacol 4:66–75, 1984

Skolnick P, Paul SM: New concepts in the neurobiology of anxiety. J Clin Psychiatry 44:12–20, 1983

Stromgren LS, Dahl J, Fjeldborg N, et al: Factors influencing seizure duration and number of seizures applied in unilateral electroconvulsive therapy. Acta Psychiatr Scand 62:158–165, 1980

Tallman JF, Paul SM, Skolnick P, et al: Receptors for the age of anxiety: pharmacology of the benzodiazepines. Science 207:274–281, 1980

Taylor CB, Kenigsberg ML, Robinson JM: A controlled comparison of relaxation and diazepam in panic disorder. J Clin Psychiatry 43:423–425, 1982

Tyrer P, Owen R: Gradual withdrawal of diazepam after long-term therapy. Lancet 1:1402–1406, 1983

Winokur A, Rickels K, Greenblatt DJ, et al: Withdrawal reaction from long-term low-dosage administration of diazepam. Arch Gen Psychiatry 37:101–105, 1980

3

Psychopharmacology Consultation for Bulimia and Anorexia Nervosa: A Clinical Overview

David C. Jimerson, M.D.

3

Psychopharmacology Consultation for Bulimia and Anorexia Nervosa: A Clinical Overview

Although anorexia nervosa and exogenous obesity have been recognized for some time as distinctive medical syndromes with major psychological components, the identification of a distinct syndrome characterized predominantly by binge eating episodes is much more recent. Early descriptions of this syndrome included articles by Boskind-Lodahl and White (1978), Russell (1979), Palmer (1979), and Crisp (1981). The recognition of bulimia as a distinct psychiatric syndrome has resulted in increased awareness of the frequency of binge eating in young women in the population at large, and particularly in patients seeking psychiatric outpatient treatment.

The focus of this chapter is on special problems involved in psychopharmacology consultations with patients with bulimic disorder and anorexia nervosa, particularly bulimia because of its relatively recent description and greater prevalence compared with anorexia.

This research was performed by the author in his capacity as an employee of the National Institute of Mental Health and is in the public domain.

DIAGNOSIS OF BULIMIC DISORDER AND
ANOREXIA NERVOSA

In the *Diagnostic and Statistical Manual of Mental Disorders (Third Edition) (DSM-III;* American Psychiatric Association 1980) bulimia was defined as a distinct nosological entity characterized by recurrent episodes of binge eating. Eating binges are identified as the inconspicuous ingestion of a large amount of food in a discrete period of time, usually less than two hr. Preferred foods for a binge are typically sweet or salty carbohydrates, including large amounts of snack foods such as ice cream, potato chips, cake, or chocolates. Clinical reports and survey data suggest that an average binge episode ranges from 3,000 to 5,000 calories and often occurs when the patient is alone during the evening (Johnson et al. 1982; Mitchell and Laine 1985; Pyle et al. 1981). Binge episodes are typically terminated by abdominal pain, sleep, social interruption, or self-induced vomiting. Bulimic subjects are generally preoccupied with their body weight and try repeatedly to lose weight with severely restrictive diets, self-induced vomiting, or by using cathartics or diuretics. Binge episodes in bulimia are accompanied by depressed mood, self-deprecating thoughts, and an awareness that the pattern of binge eating is abnormal.

Two major diagnostic changes in the description of bulimic disorder have been proposed for the revised edition of *DSM-III.* In the original criteria of 1980 (Table 1), no minimal frequency of bulimic episodes was required, although many researchers and clinicians used a cutoff of at least one bulimic episode per week for some sustained period of time. In the proposed revised criteria, a frequency of two binges per week sustained for at least three months is required for the diagnosis.

The second major proposed change is that a concurrent diagnosis of anorexia nervosa would be permitted in conjunction with bulimic disorder. As noted previously, according to *DSM-III* criteria, patients with anorexia nervosa should not be diagnosed as having "bulimia." In practice, however, clinical reports and research surveys indicate that 30 to 50 percent of low-weight patients with anorexia nervosa engage in frequent binge eating episodes

(Casper et al. 1980; Crisp 1980; Garfinkel and Garner 1982), in contrast to the purely "restrictive" dietary pattern typical of other anorexic patients. Bulimic anorexic patients appear to share a number of psychological characteristics with normal-weight patients with bulimia, including frequent depressive symptoms, impulsive behavior, and drug abuse, as well as a previous history of wide fluctuations in body weight (Garner et al. 1985). Symptoms of disordered, idiosyncratic eating pattern are present in approximately one-half of anorexic patients after restoration to a normal body weight (Hsu 1980). It is not uncommon therefore to encounter patients who have current symptoms of bulimia and a past history of anorexia. Further research is needed to clarify whether bulimic anorexic patients are more similar to "restricting" anorexic subjects or to normal-weight patients with bulimia, from both psychological and biological perspectives.

The diagnosis of anorexia nervosa focuses on the patient's intense fear of becoming obese, a symptom that does not diminish as weight loss progresses to severe malnutrition. Body image is distorted, with a perception of looking and feeling fat, even at low weights. By definition the patient refuses to maintain weight over a minimal normal for age and height, which in *DSM-III* was set at a weight loss of at least 25 percent below original body weight. According to the proposed revised criteria for *DSM-III-R*, the weight deficit would change to a loss of at least 15 percent below expected body weight, with the additional criterion of amenorrhea for at least three months included. As for bulimia, there would be no known physical illness to account for the eating disorder.

From the standpoint of clinical evaluation of a patient with eating disorders, several additional factors need to be emphasized. Thus, even with the increasing recognition of the widespread prevalence of bulimia, diagnosis of the syndrome in an individual patient may depend on explicit inquiry about the patient's weight history and dietary patterns. This is different from the usual consultation with an anorexic patient, where the low weight is relatively apparent, and is usually identified as the reason that family, friends, or the physician or psychotherapist has recommended the consultation. It is not uncommon for a bulimic patient to report a presenting complaint of depression, situational anxiety, or problems in social relationships. If the clinician fails to inquire directly about bulimic symptoms, the patient may be reluctant to mention them until later in the treatment.

In the evaluation and treatment of a patient presenting with an identified problem with anorexia nervosa or bulimia, it is essential for the clinician to take a thorough psychiatric history including past and present symptoms of affective illness, anxiety disorders, personality disorder, and substance abuse. These syndromes occur more frequently in anorexic and bulimic patients, possibly because of shared psychobiological alterations. It is also essential to take a thorough medical history in eating disorder patients, to rule out the possibility that symptoms may be related to a medical disorder. Results of a recent physical examination and screening laboratory tests should be reviewed. There is evidence, for example, that there may be an increased frequency of bulimic behavior in diabetic patients (Rodin et al. 1985). As noted below, fasting and bulimic behaviors can result in medical complications requiring evaluation and treatment.

EPIDEMIOLOGY OF BULIMIA AND ANOREXIA NERVOSA

As one might anticipate with a recently recognized syndrome, the population lifetime prevalence of bulimia is poorly documented. Although some research reports and articles in the popular press suggest that the prevalence of bulimia has increased dramatically over the past 30 years, these observations may be skewed by past inattentiveness of clinicians to pathology in eating behaviors. Moreover, with spreading recognition of the prevalence of eating disorders, subjects with bulimia have undoubtedly become more open in seeking professional help for their symptoms. Factors that may contribute to an increasing prevalence of bulimia include increased cultural idealization of slenderness in women, increased attention to dietary selection of "healthy" (for example, low-salt, low-fat) foods, and increased stress associated with social role choices confronting young women.

Survey data from subjects seeking information on eating disorders suggest that the average age of onset of bulimia is 18 years (Fairburn and Cooper 1982; Johnson et al. 1982; Pyle et al. 1981). Onset of binge eating is usually preceded by lengthy periods of preoccupation with body weight, including frequent episodes of dieting to maintain a normal or low-normal weight. After a period of weeks to months of episodic binge eating, many subjects turn to regular postbinge self-induced vomiting as they continue to struggle with stabilizing their body weight.

Surveys of high school and college age subjects indicate a prevalence of bulimia of approximately five percent in these young women, with *DSM-III* criteria modified to require a frequency of binge episodes of at least once per week (Cooper and Fairburn 1983; Johnson et al. 1984a, 1984b; Pope et al. 1984; Pyle et al. 1983). Limited data suggest that the prevalence in men is about one tenth that observed in women. The frequency of binge-associated self-induced vomiting is approximately 20 percent in surveys of high school and college age women who meet criteria for bulimia. In other surveys, however, subjects identifying themselves as having an eating disorder frequently report binge eating on a daily basis, with a 60–85-percent incidence of associated vomiting behavior (Johnson et al. 1982; Pyle et al. 1981). The frequency of reported laxative abuse for weight control in bulimic subjects is variable but lower than the frequency of self-induced vomiting. Clinical experience suggests that frequent laxative and diuretic abuse in bulimic patients is associated with more extensive psychopathology.

The epidemiology of anorexia nervosa is more clearly established than that of bulimic disorder, with an estimated prevalence of one-half to two percent in high school and college-age women (Crisp et al. 1976; Jones et al. 1980). Nonetheless, because of the low prevalence of this syndrome in the population at large, more precise details including the socioeconomic and ethnic backgrounds of affected persons are not well established. As for bulimia, it occurs predominantly (10:1 to 20:1) in women versus men. The mean age of onset for anorexia is also 18 years. Initial suggestions that early onset was associated with better prognosis have recently been questioned (Hawley 1985).

RELATIONSHIP TO AFFECTIVE ILLNESS

Symptoms of depression are commonly reported by patients with bulimia as well as by those with anorexia nervosa (especially bulimic anorexic patients). Chronic or recurring symptoms of depression are often the presenting complaint in bulimic subjects seeking outpatient treatment. Using formal diagnostic criteria, several authors have reported a high frequency of present or past episodes of affective illness in bulimic patients, with estimates ranging from 60 to 88 percent (Gwirtsman et al. 1983; Hudson et al. 1982, 1983c; Walsh et al. 1985a). Estimates of the prevalence of major depression or bipolar disorder in bulimic patients are more variable, although still high (17–75 percent) (Gwirtsman et al. 1983; Herzog 1982; Hudson et al. 1983c; Walsh et al. 1985a). Further evidence for a connection between bulimia and affective illness has been reported in family studies demonstrating a high lifetime prevalence of affective illness in relatives of bulimics. Hudson et al. (1983a) reported that 16.3 percent of first-degree relatives of bulimic subjects had a history of major depression or bipolar illness, a figure similar to that obtained for families of probands with affective illness, but significantly higher than other psychiatric control groups.

As noted above, bulimic patients frequently describe recurring symptoms of situational depression, as well as anxiety, and these often seem to be the immediate trigger for an episode of bingeing and vomiting (Abraham and Beumont 1982; Johnson and Larson 1982; Mitchell et al. 1985; Weiss and Ebert 1983). Subjective reports have yielded mixed opinions on the possible efficacy of binge/vomiting episodes in relieving these symptoms. Results of a recent study at the National Institute of Mental Health (NIMH) showed a significant reduction in anxiety ratings after a binge episode, with little alteration in depression ratings (Kaye et al. in press).

The prevalence of present or past episodes of affective syndromes is also high in patients with anorexia nervosa (Gershon et al. 1984; Hudson et al. 1983a, 1983c). A substantial number of these patients have depressive episodes preceding the onset of weight loss, suggesting that depressive symptoms in these patients are not merely a result of metabolic and neurochemical changes associated with malnutrition. Based on family interviews, a significantly increased prevalence of affective illness in families of anorexic patients has been reported in comparison with results in healthy controls. Although the data on families of bulimic patients has not yet been replicated in a study using family interviews, the present data indicate that bulimic patients and anorexic subjects may share with affectively ill patients a common underlying biological diathesis.

Evidence for a biological link between eating disorders and affective disorders also derives from data on parallel responses to neuroendocrine challenges and binge-suppressing effects of antidepressant drugs.

PSYCHOBIOLOGY OF EATING DISORDERS: CLINICAL IMPLICATIONS

Biological studies of bulimic subjects are emerging rapidly, in line with the growing awareness of the prevalence and morbidity associated with this syndrome. Studies reported to date have focused particularly on neuroendocrine, neurotransmitter, and sleep electrophysiology tests reported to be abnormal in patients with major depression.

The dexamethasone suppression test (DST) is a useful research test for identifying a relatively high percentage of patients with major depression (approximately 50 percent) with substantial overactivity of the hypothalamic–pituitary–adrenal axis. Nonsuppression on the DST is not specific to major depression, however, as similar abnormalities may be observed in other neuropsychiatric disorders, such as alcoholism and Alzheimer's disease. Nonsuppression on the DST has been observed in 35–66 percent of bulimic subjects (Gwirtsman et al. 1983; Hudson et al. 1983b; Lindy et al. 1985). The role of recent weight loss as a contributor to altered biological responses—such as on the DST—in depressed patients is a subject of some uncertainty at present. Both Gwirtsman et al. (1983) and Hudson et al. (1983b) found weak positive relationships between body weight and DST nonsuppression in bulimia. Because of uncertainty about the effects of recent bingeing and vomiting on this test, our group has studied hospitalized bulimic subjects abstinent from bingeing and vomiting for at least four weeks (Gwirtsman et al. 1986, manuscript in preparation). Preliminary results indicate approximately a 50-percent incidence of nonsuppression on the DST in bulimia under these carefully controlled conditions.

In patients with major depression, thyroid-stimulating hormone (TSH) response to thyrotropin-releasing hormone (TRH) is frequently blunted. Preliminary reports suggest that the TSH response to TRH may also be blunted in some bulimic subjects (Gwirtsman et al. 1983). In contrast, however, bulimic patients do not appear to have the shortened rapid eye movement (REM) latency generally observed in sleeping EEG recordings from depressed patients (Walsh et al. 1985b; Weilburg et al. 1985).

Future studies on the psychobiology of bulimia can be guided by previous results in depressive disorders, and by results of studies of eating behavior in animals. Although an animal model for the syndrome of bulimia is not presently available, numerous studies have shown that brain neurotransmitters, including serotonin, norepinephrine, and dopamine, play important roles in regulating eating behavior. Thus, a recent study of neuroendocrine responses to L-tryptophan in bulimic subjects suggests that these patients may have decreased activity in the hypothalamic serotonin system mediating satiety (Jimerson et al. 1986). Similarly, neuromodulators such as γ-amino butyric acid (GABA) and brain peptides such as corticotropin-releasing factor (CRF) and cholecystokinin (CCK) have important influences on eating behavior in laboratory animals. Careful assessment of neurotransmitter, neuropeptide, and neuroendocrine function in bulimia may help to identify biological vulnerabilities to this disorder.

Extensive studies have shown dysregulation of a number of endocrine systems in anorexia nervosa, including the hypothalamic–pituitary–adrenal, hypothalamic–pituitary–gonadal, and thyroid axes (Brown 1983). Some of these changes—such as hypercortisolism and reduced blood levels of triiodothyronine—are observed in starvation per se, and may be nonspecific findings in anorexia. Conversely, some of these endocrine/metabolic changes may have a specific association with the illness, as suggested (for example) by the observation that a number of anorexic women become amenorrheic prior to the onset of weight loss. Current studies are focusing on identifying clinical correlates of the alterations in norepinephrine (Gross et al. 1979; Kaye et al. 1985) and serotonin (Kaye et al. 1984) function reported in anorexia.

MEDICAL ASSESSMENT OF EATING DISORDER PATIENTS

Patients presenting with eating disorders should have a careful medical history and laboratory profile performed. In rare cases, an eating disorder may be a prominent complaint in neurological disorders, such as certain brain tumors, temporal lobe epilepsy, Kleine-Levin syndrome, or increased intracranial pressure (Krahn and Mitchell 1984). Similarly, the clinician evaluating a patient with altered eating patterns, particularly in association with weight loss, should initially include such medical conditions as hyperthyroidism, diabetes mellitus, infection, and malignancy in the differential diagnosis.

The more common medical concerns in a patient with bulimia are related to the metabolic consequences of frequent vomiting, laxative abuse, and diuretic abuse. The most common abnormalities are metabolic alkalosis, hypokalemia, and hypochloremia (Harris 1983; Lippe 1983; Pyle et al. 1981). Electrolyte abnormalities may produce fatigue and muscle weakness as well as a predisposition to cardiac arrhythmias, and must be evaluated particularly carefully in relation to pharmacotherapy. Erosion of dental enamel and parotid gland enlargement are also frequently observed. Other medical problems such as edema and gastric dilation have been reported rarely.

The possible consequences of malnutrition per se must be evaluated in bulimic patients as well as in those with anorexia. Although severe weight loss is not present in bulimia, idiosyncratic dietary habits are the rule. A careful nutritional history is an important aspect of the initial assessment of the bulimic patient.

In anorexic patients, anemia is a common finding and some very low-weight patients have received blood transfusions, although the associated hazards need careful consideration. Bradycardia and hypotension are observed in low-weight patients, and there is an increased risk of serious cardiac arrhythmias. Serum triiodothyronine (T_3) levels are reduced, with an accompanying increase in reverse T_3; these chemical indices of hypothyroidism revert to normal with weight gain.

TREATMENT: PSYCHOLOGICAL APPROACHES

Assessment of psychotherapeutic treatment approaches to bulimia needs to be made cautiously, given the limited number of controlled studies, the short follow-up periods in the available studies, and the clinical heterogeneity of bulimic patients seeking treatment. Further work is needed in evaluating the frequency of bingeing, laxative and diuretic use, as well as the severity of affective and anxiety components as predictors of treatment outcome. Thus in pharmacological trials, the response rate for bulimic symptoms in the placebo control groups has been reported to range from virtually none (Pope et al. 1983) to 50 percent (Mitchell and Groat 1984).

Psychotherapeutic outpatient treatments have most commonly centered on behavioral, cognitive, psychodynamic, and group approaches. Substantial treatment success has been reported for these different modalities, as illustrated rather dramatically by one report of complete cessation of binge eating in 24 out of 30 patients treated with a combined individual and group approach (Lacey 1983). The overall effectiveness of the psychotherapeutic approaches has recently been reviewed (Johnson et al. 1984b; Pyle et al. 1984). Again, however, the methodological limitations of these studies require caution in interpreting the results.

Psychotherapeutic approaches to anorexia have been extensively reviewed (Garner and Garfinkel 1985), with substantial emphasis on the value of cognitive-behavioral and family treatment approaches. Hospitalization is necessary when patients reach medically unstable low weights, and a cyclic pattern of readmissions to weight gain programs is not uncommon for many patients. There are a number of advantages if low-weight patients can be admitted to a specialized eating disorder treatment program, as contingency management refeeding programs require extensive staff training in the commonly used behavioral treatment approaches.

PHARMACOLOGICAL TREATMENT OF BULIMIA

Therapeutic trials of antidepressant drugs in bulimia were prompted by the clinical similarities between bulimic and depressed patients noted previously—including depressive symptoms, a family history of depression in first-degree relatives, and responses to neuroendocrine challenge tests. Because of the varying response to placebo in the controlled studies, and because of the high response rate reported in some studies of psychotherapy alone, evaluations of drug efficacy in bulimia need to rest on the limited number of controlled, double-blind studies reported to date.

The clinical efficacy of tricyclic antidepressants and the monoamine oxidase inhibitor (MAOI) phenelzine have been demonstrated in bulimia under double-blind conditions. Pope et al. (1983) reported moderate or marked decreases in binge frequency in eight of nine chronically bulimic women studied in a double-blind trial with imipramine. In the comparison group of 10 patients treated with placebo, only 1 person showed (moderate) improvement. Reduction in binge eating was significantly correlated with decreases in depression ratings in the patients treated with imipramine. Clinical improvement during drug treatment was generally sustained at follow-up (one to eight months). In a similar vein, Hughes et al. (1986) demonstrated marked improvement in 15 of 22 bulimic patients studied in a double-blind trial with desipramine.

A more cautious note on antidepressant efficacy comes from the recent study of amitriptyline by Mitchell and Groat (1984). They reported that the 72-percent reduction in the number of binge eating episodes per week observed in the drug treatment group was not significantly higher than the 52-percent reduction observed in the group treated with placebo. The reason for the high response rate in the placebo group was unexplained, as the only other treatment during the study was a minimal behavioral treatment program. Amitriptyline did have a significant antidepressant effect in the drug treatment group, although for both drug- and placebo-treated groups, reduction in bulimic symptoms was most marked in those subjects with lower depression scores at the beginning of the study. In a recent retrospective study of 22 bulimic patients treated with antidepressants, Brotman et al. (1984) also noted a dissociation between antidepressant and binge-suppression medication effects.

Walsh and co-workers (1984) have recently confirmed in a double-blind study their previous observations (1982) on the efficacy of phenelzine in bulimic patients. They reported substantial improvement in all nine patients treated with the drug, in comparison with a modest response in only two of the placebo group. Promising results with other antidepressants (Gwirtsman et al. 1984) and lithium (Hsu 1984) have been reported in uncontrolled studies, although the only double-blind study of mianserin (Sabine et al. 1983) showed no treatment effect.

In relation to the increased incidence of EEG abnormalities reported in some bulimic patients, a number of authors have studied therapeutic responses to anticonvulsant drugs in bulimia. In a double-blind trial, Wermuth and co-workers (1977) observed a significant treatment effect of phenytoin on binge frequency, but the therapeutic response was not correlated with the presence of pretreatment EEG abnormalities. Kaplan and colleagues (1983) reported significant clinical improvement in only one of six bulimic patients treated with carbamazepine.

Several potential clinical problems merit special attention in pharmacological treatment of bulimic patients. Patient compliance in taking medication, which is a significant concern in treatment nonresponders in general, requires particular attention in bulimic patients because of their commonly associated impulsivity. In antidepressant nonresponders, measurement of drug blood level by a reliable laboratory will help uncover cases of poor compliance (or rapid drug metabolism). Antidepressant-induced, weight gain can be a limiting side effect in the use of these drugs for some patients with depression. Whereas one would expect bulimic patients to be particularly alert to, and distressed by, drug-induced weight gain, this has not been a major problem in the studies reported to date. It is important to note that bulimic patients may have a high rate of placebo response in some settings (Mitchell et al. 1984), and early apparent relapse from drug response may actually be relapse from a placebo effect. Patients may also try to please their therapist or psychopharmacologist by under-reporting the frequency of bulimic episodes. Preliminary studies suggest that recurrent binge/vomiting cycles result in sustained elevation of serum amylase levels in bulimic patients (Gwirtsman et al. 1986), raising the possibility that a spot-check of serum amylase could provide a useful index of recent bulimic episodes.

PHARMACOLOGICAL TREATMENT OF ANOREXIA NERVOSA

Questions arising in pharmacological consultations with anorexic patients are related to four main problem areas: weight restoration programs for low-weight anorexics; weight maintenance programs for recently weight-recovered patients; treatment of associated psychiatric symptoms, especially depression and anxiety; and approaches to physical symptoms.

Efforts to demonstrate efficacy of medications in weight restoration programs for anorexia have been largely unsuccessful. One methodological problem in the medication trials is that they have been conducted primarily in the context of hospital treatment programs in combination with various behavioral and psychotherapeutic approaches, which are in themselves relatively successful in helping patients achieve weight gain, usually in the range of 1.5 kg/week. In controlled trials, antidepressants and neuroleptics have not been superior to placebo in advancing weight gain (Beiderman et al. 1985; Gwirtsman et al. 1984). Lithium was of some benefit in one controlled trial (Gross et al. 1981), although only a small number of patients were studied and there were confounding variables regarding the admission weights of the drug and placebo groups. Some evidence supports the efficacy of the serotonin/histamine antagonist cyproheptadine (Gwirtsman et al. 1984; Halmi et al. 1986). Recently published data from a relatively large collaborative trial found that cyproheptadine in a dose of 32 mg/day significantly improved weight gain for restrictor anorexics, although there was evidence for a detrimental drug effect in bulimic anorexics (Halmi et al. 1986). There are very few controlled data on the efficacy of drug treatment in weight maintenance treatment programs, despite the frequent relapses to low body weight experienced by a substantial number of anorexic patients.

In clinical practice, the appropriateness of medications in the treatment of anorexic patients is often determined by accompanying psychiatric symptoms. Antidepressant medications may be helpful with the depressive symptoms experienced by many anorexics. Symptoms of anxiety, including panic attacks, may be helped by treatment with minor tranquilizers or antidepressant drugs.

Medication side effects can be a significant problem in treating anorexic patients, and considerable caution is advised in patients at very low body weights. Hypotension, constipation, and cardiac side effects can be especially serious in these patients. Careful monitoring of blood chemistries and electrolytes, especially in patients with bulimic symptoms, is important.

The endocrine and other physiological alterations associated with anorexia are largely reversed with weight restoration, although return to normal function in these systems may regularly require several months after the return to a normal weight range. Thus, the chemical hypothyroidism (low T_3), hypercortisolism, and anemia of anorexia usually do not require specific medical intervention other than weight restoration. Anemia associated with iron deficiency should be treated, although patients may be resistant to taking iron supplements. Gastrointestinal symptoms are associated with the delayed gastric emptying found in anorexia, and may be partially relieved with metoclopramide (Reglan).

OVERVIEW

Psychotherapy and behavioral treatment appear to offer substantial benefit to bulimic patients. For nondepressed bulimic patients, an initial trial of psychological treatment alone should be considered. For nonresponders, the addition of antidepressant treatment in combination with psychotherapeutic/behavioral treatment should be considered. For anorexic patients, behavioral and psychotherapeutic approaches are the mainstay of refeeding and weight maintenance programs.

The available data from double-blind trials suggest that tricyclic and MAOI antidepressant drugs may help reduce the frequency of binge eating in bulimic subjects. On the other hand, treatment of bulimic patients with these drugs requires careful clinical evaluation and monitoring because of increased drug toxicity in patients with symptom-related metabolic and electrolyte abnormalities. Because of the impulsiveness of many bulimic patients, their ability to follow a low-tyramine diet must be carefully assessed prior to considering MAOI treatment. Medication approaches in anorexic patients can be important for associated symptomatology, including depression and anxiety, and there is some evidence for the efficacy of drugs (for example, cyproheptadine) in anorexia.

REFERENCES

Abraham SF, Beumont PJV: How patients describe bulimia or binge eating. Psychol Med 12:625–635, 1982

Biederman J, Herzog DB, Rivinus TM, et al: Amitriptyline in the treatment of anorexia nervosa: a double-blind, placebo-controlled study. J Clin Psychopharmacol 5:10–16, 1985

Boskind-Lodahl M, White WC: The definition and treatment of bulimarexia in college women—a pilot study. J Am Coll Health Assoc 27:84–97, 1978

Brotman AW, Herzog DB, Woods SW: Antidepressant treatment of bulimia: the relationship between bingeing and depressive symptomatology. J Clin Psychiatry 45:7–9, 1984

Brown GM: Endocrine alterations in anorexia nervosa, in Anorexia Nervosa: Recent Developments in Research. Edited by Darby PL, Garfinkel PE, Garner DM, et al. New York, Liss, 1983

Casper RC, Eckert ED, Halmi KA, et al: Bulimia: its incidence and clinical significance in patients with anorexia nervosa. Arch Gen Psychiatry 37:1030–1035, 1980

Cooper PJ, Fairburn CG: Binge-eating and self-induced vomiting in the community: a preliminary study. Br J Psychiatry 142:139–144, 1983

Crisp AH: Anorexia Nervosa: Let Me Be. London, Academic Press, 1980

Crisp AH: Anorexia nervosa at a normal weight. The abnormal weight control syndrome. Int J Psychiatry Med 11:203–234, 1981

Crisp AH, Palmer RL, Kalucy RS: How common is anorexia nervosa? Br J Psychiatry 128:549–554, 1976

Fairburn CG, Cooper PJ: Self-induced vomiting and bulimia nervosa: an undetected problem. Br Med J 284:1153–1155, 1982

Garfinkel PE, Garner DM: Anorexia Nervosa: A Multidimensional Perspective. New York, Brunner/Mazel, 1982

Garner DM, Garfinkel PE (eds): Handbook of Psychotherapy for Anorexia Nervosa and Bulimia. New York, Guilford Press, 1985

Garner DM, Garfinkel PE, O'Shaughnessy M: The validity of the distinction between bulimia with and without anorexia nervosa. Am J Psychiatry 142:581–587, 1985

Gershon ES, Schreiber JL, Hamovit JR, et al: Clinical findings in patients with anorexia nervosa and affective illness in their relatives. Am J Psychiatry 141:1419–1422, 1984

Gross HA, Lake CR, Ebert MH, et al: Catecholamine metabolism in primary anorexia nervosa. J Clin Endocrinol Metab 49:805–809, 1979

Gross HA, Ebert MH, Faden VB, et al: A double-blind controlled trial of lithium carbonate in primary anorexia nervosa. J Clin Psychopharmacol 1:376–381, 1981

Gwirtsman HE, Roy-Byrne P, Yager J, et al: Neuroendocrine abnormalities in bulimia. Am J Psychiatry 140:559–563, 1983

Gwirtsman HE, Kaye W, Weintraub M, et al: Pharmacologic treatment of eating disorders. Psychiatr Clin North Am 7:863–878, 1984

Gwirtsman HE, Yager J, Gillard BK, et al: Serum amylase and its isoenzymes in normal weight bulimia. International Journal of Eating Disorders 5:355-361, 1986

Halmi KA, Eckert E, LaDu TJ, et al: Anorexia nervosa: treatment efficacy of cyproheptadine and amitriptyline. Arch Gen Psychiatry 43:177–181, 1986

Harris RT: Bulimarexia and related serious eating disorders with medical complications. Ann Intern Med 99:800–807, 1983

Hawley RM: The outcome of anorexia nervosa in younger subjects. Br J Psychiatry 146:657–660, 1985

Herzog DB: Bulimia in the adolescent. Am J Dis Child 136:985–989, 1982

Hsu LKG: Outcome of anorexia nervosa: a review of the literature (1954 to 1978). Arch Gen Psychiatry 37:1041–1046, 1980

Hsu LKG: Treatment of bulimia with lithium. Am J Psychiatry 141:1260–1262, 1984

Hudson JI, Laffer PS, Pope HG Jr: Bulimia related to affective disorder by family history and response to the dexamethasone suppression test. Am J Psychiatry 139:685–687, 1982

Hudson JI, Pope HG Jr., Jonas JM, et al: Family history study of anorexia nervosa and bulimia. Br J Psychiatry 142:133–138, 1983a

Hudson JI, Pope HG Jr, Jonas JM, et al: Hypothalamic–pituitary–adrenal axis hyperactivity in bulimia. Psychiatry Res 8:111–117, 1983b

Hudson JI, Pope HG Jr., Jonas JM, et al: Phenomenologic relationship of eating disorder to major affective disorder. Psychiatry Res 9:345–354, 1983c

Hughes PL, Wells LA, Cunningham CJ, et al: Treating bulimia with desipramine: a double-blind, placebo-controlled study. Arch Gen Psychiatry 43:182–186, 1986

Jimerson DC, Brewerton TD, George DT, et al: Neurotransmitter function and symptom profiles in bulimia, in Biological Psychiatry 1985. Edited by Shagass C, Josiassen RC, Bridger WH, et al. New York, Elsevier, 1986

Johnson C, Larson R: Bulimia: an analysis of moods and behavior. Psychosom Med 44:341–351, 1982

Johnson CL, Stuckey MK, Lewis LD, et al: Bulimia: a descriptive survey of 316 cases. International Journal of Eating Disorders 2:3–18, 1982

Johnson CL, Lewis C, Love S, et al: Incidence and correlates of bulimic behavior in a female high school population. Journal of Youth and Adolescence 13:15–26, 1984a

Johnson CL, Lewis C, Hagman J: The syndrome of bulimia: review and synthesis. Psychiatr Clin North Am 7:247–273, 1984b

Jones DJ, Fox MM, Babigian HM, et al: Epidemiology of anorexia nervosa in Monroe County, New York: 1960–1976. Psychosom Med 42:551–558, 1980

Kaplan AS, Garfinkel PE, Darby PL, et al: Carbamazepine in the treatment of bulimia. Am J Psychiatry 140:1225–1226, 1983

Kaye WH, Ebert MH, Gwirtsman HE, et al: Differences in brain serotonergic metabolism between nonbulimic and bulimic patients with anorexia nervosa. Am J Psychiatry 141:1598–1601, 1984

Kaye WH, Jimerson DC, Lake CR, et al: Altered norepinephrine metabolism following long-term weight recovery in patients with anorexia nervosa. Psychiatry Res 14:333–342, 1985

Kaye WH, Gwirtsman HE, George DT, et al: Relationship of mood alterations to bingeing behavior in bulimia. Br J Psychiatry, in press

Krahn DD, Mitchell JE: Case report of bulimia associated with increased intracranial pressure. Am J Psychiatry 141:1099–1100, 1984

Lacey JH: Bulimia nervosa, binge eating and psychogenic vomiting: a controlled treatment study and long term outcome. Br Med J 186:1609–1613, 1983

Lindy DC, Walsh BT, Roose SP, et al: The dexamethasone suppression test in bulimia. Am J Psychiatry 142:1372–1376, 1985

Lippe BM: The physiologic aspects of eating disorders. J Am Acad Child Psychiatry 22:108–113, 1983

Mitchell JE, Groat R: A placebo-controlled, double-blind trial of amitriptyline in bulimia. J Clin Psychopharmacol 4:186–193, 1984

Mitchell JE, Laine DC: Monitored binge-eating behavior in patients with bulimia. International Journal of Eating Disorders 4:177–183, 1985

Mitchell JE, Hatsukami D, Eckert ED, et al: Characteristics of 275 patients with bulimia. Am J Psychiatry 142:482–485, 1985

Palmer RL: The dietary chaos syndrome: a useful new term? Br J Med Psychol 52:187–190, 1979

Pope HG Jr, Hudson JI, Jonas JM, et al: Bulimia treated with imipramine: a placebo-controlled, double-blind study. Am J Psychiatry 140:554–558, 1983

Pope HG Jr., Hudson JI, Yurgelun-Todd D: Anorexia nervosa and bulimia among 300 suburban women shoppers. Am J Psychiatry 141:292–294, 1984

Pyle RL, Mitchell JE, Eckert ED: Bulimia: a report of 34 cases. J Clin Psychiatry 42:60–64, 1981

Pyle RL, Mitchell JE, Eckert ED, et al: The incidence of bulimia in freshman college students. International Journal of Eating Disorders 2:75–85, 1983

Pyle RL, Mitchell JE, Eckert ED: The interruption of bulimic behaviors: a review of three treatment programs. Psychiatr Clin North Am 7:275–286, 1984

Rodin GM, Daneman D, Johnson LE, et al: Anorexia nervosa and bulimia in female adolescents with insulin dependent diabetes mellitus: a systematic study. J Psychiatr Res 19:381–384, 1985

Russell G: Bulimia nervosa: an ominous variant of anorexia nervosa. Psychol Med 9:429–448, 1979

Sabine EJ, Yonace A, Farrington AJ, et al: Bulimia nervosa: a placebo controlled double-blind therapeutic trial of mianserin. Br J Clin Pharmacol 15:195S–202S, 1983

Walsh BT, Stewart JW, Wright L, et al: Treatment of bulimia with monoamine oxidase inhibitors. Am J Psychiatry 139:1629–1630, 1982

Walsh BT, Stewart JW, Roose SP, et al: Treatment of bulimia with phenelzine: a double-blind, placebo-controlled study. Arch Gen Psychiatry 41:1105–1109, 1984

Walsh BT, Roose SP, Glassman AH, et al: Bulimia and depression. Psychosom Med 47:123–131, 1985a

Walsh BT, Goetz R, Roose SP, et al: EEG-monitored sleep in anorexia nervosa and bulimia. Biol Psychiatry 20:947–956, 1985b

Weilburg JB, Stakes JW, Brotman A, et al: Sleep architecture in bulimia: a pilot study. Biol Psychiatry 20:199–228, 1985

Weiss SR, Ebert MH: Psychological and behavioral characteristics of normal-weight bulimics and normal-weight controls. Psychosom Med 45:293–303, 1983

Wermuth BM, Davis KL, Hollister LE, et al: Phenytoin treatment of the binge-eating syndrome. Am J Psychiatry 134:1249–1253, 1977

4

Pharmacotherapeutic Approaches to Schizophrenia

David Pickar, M.D.

4

Pharmacotherapeutic Approaches to Schizophrenia

This chapter contains an overview of the pharmacotherapy of schizophrenia oriented toward problems facing the consultant. Because neuroleptic drugs (also known as antipsychotic drugs or major tranquilizers) are the most important first-line treatment for schizophrenia (and psychosis in general), they are given the most attention, with an emphasis on their clinical effects, their mechanism of action, and perspectives that may be helpful in optimizing their clinical efficacy and minimizing their untoward effects. Other drugs that have a place in the pharmacotherapy of schizophrenia are presented based on their clinical indications.

CLINICAL PERSPECTIVES

Research over the past decade includes material from biologically oriented investigators as well as from psychotherapists, sociologists, and epidemiologists that affects our understanding of schizophrenia. The lack of a clearly defined brain pathology and/or biochemical etiology in schizophrenia renders such diverse elements important to any clinician involved in the care of schizophrenic patients.

This research was performed by the author in his capacity as an employee of the National Institute of Mental Health and is in the public domain.

One of the most important contributions in recent years has been the development of readily applied diagnostic criteria, improving our ability to identify and treat a relatively homogeneous group of patients. The *Diagnostic and Statistical Manual of Mental Disorders (Third Edition)* (*DSM-III*; American Psychiatric Association 1980), influenced by the highly successful Research Diagnostic Criteria (Spitzer et al. 1975), incorporates symptomatology, degree of functioning, and course of illness in the diagnosis of schizophrenia. Although not the only diagnostic framework available (see also Strauss and Carpenter 1982; Strauss and Gift 1977), it is increasingly used worldwide. One aspect of the *DSM-III* diagnosis of schizophrenia is the requirement that symptoms last for at least six months, thus excluding individuals with acute psychotic illnesses. Whereas the pharmacotherapy of acute psychosis (schizophreniform disorder or brief reactive psychosis by *DSM-III*) often involves neuroleptic treatment, the conservative approach to diagnosing schizophrenia may help to restrict long-term neuroleptic treatment to only those in whom it is clearly required.

Clinical heterogeneity in schizophrenia has long been appreciated and is included in the *DSM-III* diagnosis as the following types: disorganized, catatonic, paranoid, and undifferentiated. These subclassifications are useful in organizing a clinical perspective of schizophrenia and in clinical research on its course and prognosis. Catatonic schizophrenia, which is diminishing in prevalence (Morrison 1974), is a particularly interesting subtype. Catatonia is defined in *DSM-III* by the presence of one of a number of elements, including severe negativism and abnormal motor activity characterized by stupor, marked rigidity, posturing, or periods of excitation. Because some of these features are also found in bipolar affective disorder (Abrams and Taylor 1976; Taylor and Abrams 1977) or in patients with organic lesions, differential diagnosis is important (see the review by Stoudemire 1982). Paranoid disorders, of which the essential features are persistent persecutory or jealousy delusions in individuals in whom the diagnosis of schizophrenia cannot be made (see the review by Kendler 1984), are a particularly difficult group of psychotic illnesses to treat pharmacologically, both because of limitations in therapeutic alliance and the refractoriness of the delusions to pharmaco-therapy. Schizoaffective illness, often considered a subtype of schizophrenia, is discussed later in the chapter.

The assessment of overall clinical state and the identification of target symptoms by clinical interview and review of historical data are the first steps in the psychopharmacological consultation pro-cess. It should be kept in mind that many of the psychotic symp-toms or behaviors characteristic of schizophrenia are in and of themselves nonspecific and can be associated with serious organic pathology. At times the distinction between organic and func-tional psychosis is difficult. The availability of computerized axial tomography (CAT) scanners in most hospitals has improved the early identification of CNS lesions and has a place in differential diagnosis in psychiatry (see the discussion by Weinberger 1984). When doubt remains concerning the presence of an organic lesion there should be no hesitation in requesting a consultation by a neurologist.

Because behavioral change in patients with schizophrenia may be gradual or subtle (particularly in patients requiring consulta-tion), a useful tool is the quantification by a rating scale of key symptoms and/or clinical state prior to and throughout treatment. Performed "blindly" in research, the "open" clinical setting should not preclude its application. The Brief Psychiatric Rating Scale (BPRS; Overall and Gorham 1961) is perhaps the most widely used rating instrument for psychotic patients; its attention to di-verse symptoms, however, may make it cumbersome in clinical practice. The clinician may find a global rating scale based on severity of target symptoms and behavioral dysfunction more practical. Table 1 shows the global rating scale for psychosis used by our research group, a modification of the Bunney-Hamburg scale (Bunney and Hamburg 1963), with "anchor" points oriented to a seriously ill population of schizophrenic patients. The fre-quency of a scale's application should be determined by the setting (such as inpatient versus outpatient), and the nature of the symp-toms to be treated; unless specific short-term change is expected, weekly ratings are sufficient.

In recent years there has been a renewed emphasis on the historical concept of "positive" and "negative" symptomatology

Table 1.   Global Ratings for Psychosis

Score	Guidelines
1–3	*Minimal, within the range of normal.* Ratings of 2 or 3 may reflect odd or strange manner, apathy, somewhat flat affect, social withdrawal, and inattention or suspiciousness.
4–6	*Mild symptoms of psychosis.* These include some distortions of reality, difficulties with logic, and instances of inappropriate affect or inappropriate interpersonal relations. Patients may rarely report hearing voices, without responding to them, or noninterfering delusions, without elaboration.
7–9	*Moderate symptoms of psychosis.* These include more evident conceptual disorganization. Some reality testing and contact with reality is maintained (such as, the patient will consider staff explanations), but the patient could not function for more than a day or two without hospitalization. Symptoms may include hallucinations throughout the day, interfering delusions, severe thought blocking, looser associations, and markedly inappropriate affect.
10–12	*Severe symptoms of psychosis.* Major loss of contact with reality. Multiple psychotic symptoms are present including definite thought disorder, pervasive involvement with hallucinations, preoccupation with very bizarre thoughts or ideas, little control over behavior, and the inability to function outside a hospital.
13–15	*Very severe symptoms of psychosis.* Absence of reality contact, with loss of ego boundaries. Multiple symptoms of psychosis are continually present, although the patient will often be sufficiently out of touch that he or she may not verbalize symptoms. Frequently characterized by catatonia, severe agitation or combativeness, smearing, or word salad. Minimal self-care is usually impossible for the patient.

Note. Adapted from the Bunney-Hamburg Scale (1963).

(see the discussion by Berrios 1985). As applied to schizophrenia, positive symptoms include delusions, hallucinations, formal thought disorder, and disorientation; negative symptoms include apathy, motor retardation, social withdrawal, and paucity of thought and communication. It has been hypothesized (Crow 1980, 1981) with some experimental support (Andreasen et al. 1982; Weinberger et al. 1980), that positive symptoms are related to overactivity of CNS dopamine systems and are neuroleptic responsive in contrast to negative symptoms, which result from a nondopamine organic pathology (possibly reflected by increased brain ventricular size on CAT scan) and respond poorly to neuroleptics. Although the importance of this hypothesis is clear, its clinical validity has not been fully tested. Furthermore, from a clinical perspective it can be difficult to distinguish a symptom such as social withdrawal, which may be part of a neuroleptic-responsive psychosis, from an enduring behavioral manifestation of schizophrenia (see the discussion by Kety 1980). An empirical drug trial is indicated even in the presence of negative symptoms or of relative enlargement of the cerebral ventricles in the absence of a neurological lesion.

FUNDAMENTALS OF NEUROLEPTIC TREATMENT

Clinical Effects

The discovery of chlorpromazine and the subsequent demonstration of its unique effectiveness in reducing symptoms of psychosis (Delay and Deniker 1952) are a landmark not only for psychiatry but for all of medicine. Many drugs from the group known as neuroleptics have been shown in double-blind controlled studies to have antipsychotic activity. Despite differing chemical structures and ranges of side effects, there is little experimental support indicating the greater effectiveness of one or another agent in the treatment of schizophrenia or specific psychotic symptoms (Goldberg et al. 1972; Hollister et al. 1974).

The truly remarkable clinical effects produced by neuroleptics may not always be appreciated by clinicians trained in the postneuroleptic era, as outside of research ward settings there is little opportunity to observe over time unmedicated, highly symptomatic schizophrenic patients and their subsequent drug response. The nature of the antipsychotic response produced by neuroleptic treatment has been documented in numerous studies (see reviews by Baldessarini 1980; Davis et al. 1983). In summary, neuroleptics improve a wide range of symptoms associated with schizophrenia, including positive symptoms such as thought disorder and hallucinations, as well as negative symptoms such as social withdrawal, poverty of thought, and autistic behavior. The course of response is classically time-dependent, with optimal effects appearing over weeks and in some cases over months. Rapid neuroleptization, suggested as a means of enhancing the rapidity of clinical response (Donlon and Tupin 1975), has little controlled experimental support, and probably provides little advantage beyond acute behavioral control (Anderson et al. 1976; Neborsky et al. 1981). Despite the fact that prolonged treatment is required for many schizophrenic patients without achieving an eventual "cure," the proven effectiveness of neuroleptics in diminishing the rate of relapse and need for hospitalization (Davis 1975; Hogarty et al. 1975) has unquestionably altered the clinical course of the illness.

Mechanism of Action

The foundation for the dopamine hypothesis of schizophrenia is based most clearly on the effects of neuroleptics on CNS dopamine systems (see the reviews by Carlsson 1978; Meltzer and Stahl 1976). The initial proposal by Carlsson and Lindquist (1963) that neuroleptic drugs produce a blockade of dopamine transmission was based on their observation of neuroleptic-induced increases in the accumulation of dopamine metabolites, suggesting a compensatory increase in dopamine release in response to transmission blockade. Numerous subsequent biochemical studies have supported this initial finding (see the review by Roth 1983). In 1973, Bunney and co-workers (1973) demonstrated a neuroleptic-induced functional increase in dopamine neuronal activity using single unit electrophysiological techniques.

The identification of the dopamine receptor or receptors by radioligand binding techniques (Iversen 1975; Kebabian et al. 1972) led to a second body of evidence closely linking dopamine blockade to antipsychotic effects. There is a close correlation among known antipsychotic agents between their milligram clinical potency and affinity for the non-adenyl cyclase-dependent dopamine receptor (D_2 receptor) in rodent brain preparations (Creese et al. 1976; Seeman et al. 1976). Although the precise anatomical location of all neuroleptic effects is not fully known, the following conceptualization represents our current understanding. The extrapyramidal side effects of neuroleptics are a result of dopamine blockade in the nigrostriatal dopamine system of the basal ganglia, and endocrine effects, such as increased secretion of prolactin, are the result of dopamine blockade in the pituitary tuberoinfundibular system. More complex dopamine systems involving projections from the midbrain to limbic and cortical regions (mesolimbic and mesocortical dopamine systems) have been hypothesized to be the sites of antipsychotic actions and possibly of the underlying dopamine pathophysiology of schizophrenia (Stevens 1973).

A limitation to the notion that blockade of dopamine transmission is directly related to antipsychotic effects is the fact that although blockade occurs rapidly after the administration of neuroleptics, clinical improvement is slow to develop. Investigators have recently examined differences between acute and chronic effects of neuroleptics on dopamine neuronal function. Whereas short-term administration produces increased dopamine neuronal firing rates in electrophysiological models, prolonged administration is associated with a markedly reduced firing rate, an effect thought to be the result of "depolarization block" (Bunney 1984; Bunney and Grace 1978; White and Wang 1983). Differences between acute and chronic neuroleptic effects have also been observed using biochemical techniques (Lerner et al. 1977; Roth et al. 1980).

In our current studies of schizophrenic patients we are using plasma levels of the dopamine metabolite homovanillic acid (HVA) to provide a reflection of dopamine turnover. We have observed a neuroleptic-induced, time-dependent decrease in levels of plasma HVA, with levels falling significantly below baseline only after three weeks of fluphenazine treatment (Pickar et al. 1984). We have further observed that this decrease in dopamine turnover, as reflected by decreases in plasma HVA, is highly correlated with the antipsychotic response of the patients. Thus, slowly developing changes in dopamine release, probably an adaptation to dopamine receptor blockade, may be more closely related to the eventual antipsychotic effect than the receptor blockade itself. This model for the mechanism of antipsychotic action may serve as a biological marker for antipsychotic response, eventually helping to predict and improve drug response in individual patients.

Adverse Effects

Although neuroleptic drugs have a high therapeutic index and are quite safe, they are associated with a number of side effects, a thorough understanding of which is important for their proper use. The spectrum of side effects of an individual neuroleptic can be predicted by the corresponding potency of blocking properties for each of the following receptor sites in the human caudate: D_2, dopamine; H_1, histamine, muscarinic, and α_1-adrenergic (Richelson 1984) (Table 2). Note that in general the more milligram-potent a drug is in producing antipsychotic effects, the more potent the agent is in producing antidopaminergic (extrapyramidal) side effects, but the less potent it is in producing antimuscarinic (dry mouth, constipation, and so on) and antihistaminic (sedation) side effects.

Extrapyramidal side effects are the most important adverse effects of neuroleptic drugs and include parkinsonism, acute dystonia, akinesis, and akathisia. They are thought to be related to antidopaminergic effects of neuroleptics in the nigrostriatal system. Table 3 contains a summary of extrapyramidal side effects and treatment approaches.

Tardive dyskinesia, the most serious of the extrapyramidal side effects, is characterized by abnormal oral–facial movements, which in severe cases may extend to the limbs and torso. It differs from other extrapyramidal side effects by being highly resistant to treatment, even neuroleptic discontinuation (see the review by Jeste and Wyatt 1979). Though hypothetically related to postsynaptic dopamine receptor supersensitivity (Baldessarini and Tarsy 1979), its pathophysiology is not yet fully understood. Because of the clear association between neuroleptic treatment and tardive dyskinesia, when the syndrome is recognized in a patient (occasionally it becomes apparent after a decrease in neuroleptic dose), an attempt should be made to manage the patient free from neuroleptics. When a neuroleptic is required, it is suggested that an "atypical" neuroleptic be used, one of several agents that are effective antipsychotics but have minimal extrapyramidal side effects. The most commonly used atypical neuroleptics are

Table 2. Side Effects of Neuroleptic Drugs Due to Receptor Blockade

Dopaminergic (D_2) blockade	Muscarinic (cholinergic) blockade	Histaminergic (H_1) blockade	Adrenergic (α_1) blockade
Extrapyramidal side effects	Dry mouth	Sedation	Orthostatic hypotension (lightheadedness)
Increased prolactin (galactorrhea, menstrual changes)	Constipation	Drowsiness	
	Sinus tachycardia	Weight gain	
	Urinary retention	Hypotension	
	Speech and memory dysfunction		
	Exacerbation of glaucoma		

Adapted from Richelson (1984).

Table 3. Summary of Neuroleptic-Induced Extrapyramidal Side Effects

Syndrome	Clinical presentation	Treatment
Acute dystonia	Spasm of muscles in face, tongue, neck or back; onset early in treatment (first week); can be confused with catatonic posturing	Antiparkinsonian agents[a] and diphenhydramine (oral or parenteral)
Parkinsonism	Bradykinesia, rigidity, tremor, masklike faces; onset most common during first weeks of treatment	Antiparkinsonian agents[a]
Akinesia	Marked decrease in motor activity and depression; resembles catatonia or psychotic regression; onset during first few weeks of treatment	Amantadine or decrease in neuroleptic dose
Akathisia	Motor restlessness frequently associated with psychological discomfort; may appear as worsening psychosis or anxiety; onset over first months of treatment	May not respond to antiparkinsonian agents[a]; propranolol reported useful; decrease dose or change in neuroleptic may be required
Tardive dyskinesia	Oral—facial dyskinesia with torso and limb choreoathetoid movements in severe cases; classically after years of treatment or unmasked by dosage decrease; reversible form may be apparent earlier in treatment	Treatment largely unsuccessful; use of "atypical" neuroleptics when continuing drug therapy is required

[a] Benztropine, trihexyphenidyl, amantadine, and so on.

thioridazine and molindone, although others are available outside of the United States. Whether they actually do not aggravate (or cause) tardive dyskinesia is not known and is in fact difficult to test. However, these drugs are unique among the neuroleptics in that they do not produce changes in nigrostriatal dopamine neuron firing rates, whereas they do produce predictable neuroleptic changes in mesolimbic dopamine cells (White and Wang 1983).

The neuroleptic malignant syndrome, a rare but life-threatening (estimated 20 percent fatal) side effect of neuroleptic treatment, is a true medical emergency and should be recognized immediately. The clinical picture includes severe hyperthermia, muscular rigidity, autonomic dysfunction, and altered consciousness with a rapid onset and a fulminant course (see reviews by Birkhimer and DeVane 1984; Caroff 1980). It reportedly occurs during treatment with a number of different neuroleptics and its occurrence is not limited to particularly high doses. Physiologically supportive therapy and immediate discontinuation of neuroleptic treatment is the crucial first step. Dopamine agonists, anticholinergic agents, and parenteral benzodiazepines may be useful in treating this condition (May et al. 1983), which even with therapy can last from several days to several weeks. The pathophysiology of neuroleptic malignant syndrome is unknown, with both central and peripheral mechanisms having been suggested (Henderson and Wosten 1981).

Choice of Neuroleptic

The choice of neuroleptic for the individual patient is largely determined by the range of an agent's side effects. When sedation is desirable, the less milligram-potent neuroleptic may be useful, although their prominent autonomic effects may limit dosage. Atypical neuroleptics are most appropriate when tardive dyskinesia is suspected. Familiarity with the full spectrum of side effects should precede the clinical use of a given drug. Regardless of choice, a therapeutic trial should involve doses in the known antipsychotic range. Table 4 shows a summary of side effects and antipsychotic dose ranges for a representative group of neuroleptics.

Table 4. Summary of Neuroleptic Dose Ranges and Side Effects

Drug (trade name)	Antipsychotic doses, mg/day (Higher Range)[a]	Equivalent to 100 mg chlorpromazine	Sedation	Anticholinergic	Extrapyramidal side effects	Hypotensive
Phenothiazines						
Chlorpromazine (Thorazine)	300–800 (2,000)	100	+++	++	++	++
Thioridazine (Mellaril)	200–600[b] (800)	100	+++	++	+[c]	++
Trifluoperazine (Stelazine)	6–20 (60)	2–5	+	+	+++	+
Perphenazine (Trilafon)	8–32 (64)	4–8	++	+	+++	+
Fluphenazine (Prolixin)	2.5–20 (30)	2–5	+	+	+++	+
Thioxanthene						
Thiothixene (Navane)	6–30 (60)	2–4	++	+	++	++
Butyrophenone						
Haloperidol (Haldol)	6–20 (100)	2–4	+	+	+++	+
Dihydroindolone						
Molindone (Moban)	50–225 (400)	10	++	+/0	+[c]	0

Note. + = mild; ++ = moderate; +++ = marked.
[a] Adapted from Baldessarini (1980).
[b] Maximum dose of 800 mg/day because of retinal side effects.
[c] Least potent neuroleptics in producing extrapyramidal side effects. Atypical neuroleptics.

Optimizing Neuroleptic Effects

Optimizing neuroleptic treatment is frequently the most important contribution of a psychopharmacological consultant. The first strategy may be to simplify an unnecessarily complex existing treatment; there is no sound justification for using more than one neuroleptic simultaneously. Drugs that may worsen psychoses, such as antidepressants, should be stopped and an adequate assessment of neuroleptic response made.

The recognition and proper treatment of extrapyramidal side effects is an important component in optimizing the therapeutic effects of neuroleptics. Although it is uncommon to find obvious signs of parkinsonism unrecognized, other extrapyramidal side effects such as akinesis and akathisia may not be fully appreciated as side effects but rather as part of the psychosis. A catatonic-like picture can be caused by severe akinesia; increasing the dose of anticholinergic agents or the addition of the mildly dopaminergic agent amantadine (100–300 mg/day) may be useful (Gelenberg and Mandel 1977). Akathisia, a uniquely uncomfortable condition, may not be particularly responsive to anticholinergic agents; success has recently been reported in treating akathisia with the β-adrenergic blocker propranolol in doses of 30–80 mg/day (Lipinski et al. 1984). When additive medications do not provide adequate relief, a decrease in drug dosage or changing to another less potent neuroleptic is indicated.

The dosage of neuroleptic is another important facet in optimizing therapeutic response. "Antipsychotic doses" of neuroleptics (Table 4) should be viewed as guidelines rather than rules. There is clear individual variability in both the dose tolerated and that required to achieve antipsychotic response. The best approach is to titrate the dose upward to a predictably antipsychotic range with side effects and behavioral response as guidelines. Blood levels of neuroleptics can be determined by assays specific for the compound and its active metabolites (often a very difficult set of procedures) or by radioreceptor assay measuring levels of circulating dopamine receptor binding potency. Examination of the now large literature attempting to relate clinical response to plasma levels of neuroleptics reveals largely disappointing results (see the review by Meltzer et al. 1983). It is thus doubtful whether the measurement of neuroleptic levels on a regular basis produces as much clinical benefit as does careful clinical titration of the drug. In cases where idiosyncratic drug metabolism or noncompliance is suggested, blood levels may be important. In the former, measurement of the specific compound and metabolites is required, whereas in the latter radioreceptor assay determination provides the desired information. When noncompliance is a factor, depot fluphenazine, a safe and effective form of treatment (Ayd 1975), should be considered.

In achieving an optimal clinical response, dose flexibility is required; standardized antipsychotic doses represent a somewhat conservative range at both the high and low ends. Relatively low doses of neuroleptic may be sufficient for long-term management once the patient has been clinically stabilized, and occasionally, low doses of neuroleptic (particularly the more potent agents) are optimal for achieving a favorable clinical outcome from the outset (Marder et al. 1979). The use of extremely high doses of neuroleptics (such as several hundred milligrams of fluphenazine or haloperidol) to treat refractory patients has been advocated (Bjorndal et al. 1980; Donlon 1976). Although controlled studies have failed to document an overall therapeutic effect (Quitkin et al. 1975; Zarifian et al. 1982), it is generally a safe procedure that interestingly is associated with little worsening in extrapyramidal side effects and may be helpful on an empirical basis.

A therapeutic trial of neuroleptic discontinuation is indicated in instances when there is doubt concerning the need for ongoing treatment. The clinical outcome of drug discontinuation may follow one of the following courses: (a) rapid psychotic decompensation, (b) transient "improvement" manifesting as more spontaneous affect and behavior or occasionally improvement in overt psychotic symptoms lasting days or weeks followed by increasing psychotic decompensation, or (c) sustained clinical improvement. When discontinuing neuroleptic treatment, alertness to early signs of decompensation (Docherty et al. 1978; Donlon and Blacker 1973) is important to avoid a severe deterioration in the clinical condition. A trial of drug discontinuation should not be confused with a "drug holiday," an unproven strategy suggested to decrease the risk of tardive dyskinesia.

TREATMENT OF NEUROLEPTIC-RESISTANT SYMPTOMATOLOGY

In an unfortunate number of schizophrenic patients, overt psychotic symptoms including hallucinations, delusions, and disorganized or regressed behavior may persist despite attempts to maximize the therapeutic effects of neuroleptics. These symptoms interfere with the patient's functioning and often result in a restrictive clinical setting. In such cases additional pharmacotherapy should be considered. Because very few schizophrenic patients show absolutely no response to neuroleptics, unless otherwise documented, agents should be added to a stabilized neuroleptic treatment regimen. The following treatments have all been shown to help some patients; none, however, has the proven effectiveness of neuroleptics.

Presynaptic Dopamine Interventions

The notion that agents that decrease the activity of presynaptic dopamine neurons are synergistic to dopamine blocking drugs is consistent with data indicating that antipsychotic effects of neuroleptics are related to decreased dopamine turnover (Pickar et al. 1984). Acute administration of apomorphine in doses that stimulate (presynaptic) autoreceptors has been observed to augment antipsychotic effects of neuroleptics in at least one study (Tamminga et al. 1978). Because of inherent difficulties in maintaining specificity during chronic administration, however, apomorphine is best used as a pharmacological probe.

Reserpine, a Rauwolfia alkaloid, not included in the earlier discussion of neuroleptics, was the first known antipsychotic agent. The profile of reserpine's clinical effects can be predicted by its major pharmacological action, the depletion of intraneuronal stores of the monoamine neurotransmitters dopamine, serotonin, and norepinephrine. Thus, reserpine is antipsychotic; it can induce depression and is an effective antihypertensive. Although the phenothiazines were first used as additive agents to reserpine (Barsa and Line 1955; Braun 1960), reserpine's use as an antipsychotic gradually was eclipsed by neuroleptic drugs. The addition of reserpine to a stabilized neuroleptic regimen may enhance the antipsychotic response in treatment-resistant patients (Bacher and Lewis 1978). Metyrosine (α-methyl-p-tyrosine), an inhibitor of tyrosine hydroxylase, the rate-limiting enzyme in catecholamine synthesis, reduces presynaptic catecholamine stores by blocking their synthesis. Willander et al. (1976) demonstrated that metyrosine potentiated thioridazine effects in chronic schizophrenic patients; a finding, however, that was not fully replicated in a subsequent independent investigation (Nasrallah et al. 1977).

The addition of one of these two agents to a neuroleptic should be undertaken conservatively and in a setting where the patient can be carefully monitored, as both agents can produce hypotensive effects, enhanced extrapyramidal side effects, possibly depression, and in the case of metyrosine, crystalluria. Reserpine should be tried first with a starting dose of 0.25 mg b.i.d. increasing to a total daily dose in the 6–8 mg range. The development of selective antidopaminergic drugs acting through presynaptic mechanisms is an important goal for future antipsychotic drugs.

Lithium

Although the best indication for lithium in the treatment of schizophrenia is in those patients with affective symptoms (see the discussion later in this chapter), a lithium trial may be indicated in refractory psychotic patients or in patients in whom neuroleptics cannot be used, such as patients with tardive dyskinesia. Despite the fact that controlled studies of lithium alone in schizophrenic patients are consistent in failing to demonstrate a significant group antipsychotic response (Alexander et al. 1979; Growe et al. 1979; Shopsin et al. 1971; Small et al. 1975), some of these studies have documented good clinical response in individual patients, including improvement in core schizophrenic symptoms (Alexander et al. 1979; Small et al. 1975; Zemlan et al. 1984). Other than clinical improvement during the first week of treatment, no good predictors of lithium response have been found, thus emphasizing the importance of an empirical trial.

Propranolol

The use of the β-adrenergic blocker propranolol in high doses (over 400 mg/day) was reported in the 1970s as a useful treatment for schizophrenia (Atsmon et al. 1972; Yorkston et al. 1974), a finding ultimately not replicated by others (Belmaker et al. 1979; Gardos et al. 1973; Peet et al. 1981). Although this literature is far from compelling, an empirical trial of it as an additive agent to neuroleptics may be worthwhile (Lindstrom and Persson 1980; Yorkston et al. 1977). Considerable care, however, should be taken because propranolol in near gram doses has significant cardiovascular effects, suggesting that its use be restricted to an inpatient setting.

Benzodiazepines

In recent years our understanding of the preclinical pharmacology of benzodiazepines has greatly increased, including the recognition of endogenous benzodiazepine receptors in the central nervous system (Skolnick and Paul 1982) and of the behavioral effects of new benzodiazepine receptor antagonists (Insel et al. 1984). Whereas the therapeutic effectiveness of benzodiazepines in schizophrenia has been shown to be minimal (see the review by Donaldson et al. 1983), the availability of newer agents has prompted recent trials. Alprazolam, a trizolobenzodiazepine, has been shown to be a unique benzodiazepine with some effectiveness in treating both depression and anxiety (Dawson et al. 1984). Alprazolam has been reported to improve schizophrenic symptomatology in an open study of concurrently neuroleptic treated schizophrenic patients (Csernansky et al. 1984). Ongoing double-blind studies on our research ward have indicated synergistic actions between alprazolam (1.5–4.0 mg/day) and neuroleptics on both positive and negative symptoms in individual patients. As recent work has shown some mesocortical dopamine neurons to be insensitive to neuroleptics but highly responsive to benzodiazepine system activation (R. Roth, personal communication, 1984), benzodiazepine-neuroleptic combinations may have some preclinical justification. In particular, this combination may be useful in preventing or minimizing stress-related exacerbations of psychosis, an important clinical problem in schizophrenia. As alprazolam has significant withdrawal effects (including the risk of seizures), patient compliance and reliability in carrying out the treatment plan must be assured.

Carbamazepine

Carbamazepine is a widely used anticonvulsant effective in treating temporal lobe epilepsy. It has become an established treatment for affective disorders and in particular bipolar patients with atypical features (Post 1982; Post et al. 1983). Several studies now indicate that it may also be useful in treating schizophrenic patients, notably those patients who are aggressive, impulsive, and/ or violent (DeVogelaer 1981; Hakolu and Laulumaa 1982; Luchins 1983; Neppe 1982). It is also reportedly useful in combination with haloperidol in treating "excited psychoses" (Klein et al. 1984). At least one study, however, has reported a carbamazepine-induced worsening in symptomatology in schizophrenia (Stevens et al. 1979). It is interesting that carbamazepine-induced improvement is not restricted to impulsivity or excitement, but may also include more typical psychotic symptoms such as thought disorder (Klein et al. 1984).

Further prospective research is needed to elucidate the range of carbamazepine's effectiveness in schizophrenia. Presently, however, it is certainly worthy of a trial in neuroleptic-resistant patients, particularly in those in whom excitation, impulsivity, or aggression is a problem. The dose range should be comparable to that used in affective disorders (Post 1982).

TREATMENT OF AFFECTIVE SYMPTOMS IN SCHIZOPHRENIA

The evaluation and treatment of affective symptoms is a difficult, yet important aspect of the management of schizophrenic patients, as these symptoms interact with many aspects of the clinical course, including compliance, need for hospitalization, and suicide attempts. Consideration is first given to schizoaffective illness and then to depressive symptoms in schizophrenic patients without a history of maniclike symptoms.

Schizoaffective Illness

Valid and reliable diagnostic criteria for schizoaffective illness have been elusive; in fact, some authors question the existence of the syndrome itself (Pope et al. 1980; Tsuang et al. 1979). The *DSM-III*, for example, lists no specific criteria for schizoaffective illness, retaining its use as a diagnostic category only when a differentiation between affective disorder and schizophrenia cannot be made. In contrast, the Research Diagnostic Criteria for schizoaffective illness emphasize the presence of core elements of both schizophrenia and mood disturbance (mania or depression), further noting differences between schizoaffective mainly schizophrenic or schizoaffective mainly depressed forms of the illness, a distinction used in research studies (Baron et al. 1982) and, in my opinion, with some clinical validity. Research focusing on the presence of affective disorder or schizophrenia in first-degree relatives has not yet proven conclusive in linking schizoaffective illness to affective disorder or to schizophrenia (Baron et al. 1982; Gershon et al. 1982; Pope et al. 1980).

Whatever the diagnostic criteria or viewpoint taken regarding this clinical syndrome, few clinicians would argue that an important group of patients requires lithium-neuroleptic treatment combinations to reduce their recurrent mood disorder symptoms (most often mania) in the presence of enduring psychosis. Although difficulties in diagnosis limit the interpretation of research studies in this area, overall it appears that lithium-neuroleptic combinations are superior to either drug alone in treating such patients (see the review by Delva and Letemendia 1982). In mainly schizophrenic schizoaffectives, the range of response to neuroleptic alone should be established before adding lithium (Mattes and Nayak 1984). Severe lithium-neuroleptic toxicity (Cohen and Cohen 1974) is extremely infrequent, although potentially synergistic behavioral effects may require that a lower dose of neuroleptic be used.

Depressive Symptomatology

Depressive symptomatology in schizophrenic patients has long been recognized and is viewed psychodynamically as part of recovery from psychosis (Bowers and Astrachan 1967; Eissler 1951; Mayer-Gross 1920; Rorn 1970). Phenomenologically "postpsychotic depression" has been characterized by motor retardation and a neurasthenic presentation (McGlashan and Carpenter 1976). In one report lithium was found useful in treating this syndrome in 6 of 11 otherwise drug-free patients (Van Kammen et al. 1980). Other studies have suggested that depressive symptomatology is not necessarily linked to the psychosis recovery phase but occurs cross-sectionally at various phases of the illness (Johnson 1981a, 1981b; Knights et al. 1979; Mandel et al. 1982). The hypothesis that depressive symptoms are a result of neuroleptic treatment has not been substantiated (Hogarty and Munetz 1984; Johnson 1981a), although the differentiation between depression and subtle EPSs may be required in some patients. Depressive symptoms are associated with higher morbidity among schizophrenic patients, including rehospitalization and suicide attempts (Roy 1981; Roy et al. 1984). Except in cases in which maniclike symptoms suggest a diagnosis of schizoaffective illness, there are no real guidelines for the diagnosis of depressive symptomatology in schizophrenic patients. The *DSM-III* criteria for major depressive episodes have been applied in patients with schizophrenia (Roy 1981; Roy et al. 1984) and may help in identifying a clinically significant depressive syndrome from emotional blunting, an important symptom in schizophrenic patients (Abrams and Taylor 1978).

There is virtually no indication for the use of antidepressant medications as a sole treatment for schizophrenic patients. Some evidence suggests that antidepressant-neuroleptic combinations (tricyclic or monoamine oxidase inhibitor) may be useful in treating schizophrenic patients with depressive symptoms. Much of this evidence, however, is derived from early uncontrolled studies (see the review by Siris et al. 1978). Two recent controlled investigations of treating depressed schizophrenic outpatients with antidepressants, one using a combination of perphenazine and amitriptyline (Prusoff et al. 1979) and the other fluphenazine and nortriptyline (Johnson 1981a) are representative of the results seen in this area. One study (Prusoff et al. 1979) found significant improvement in depressed symptoms but less therapeutic improvement in thought disorder when combined treatment was compared with neuroleptic treatment alone. The other study (Johnson 1981c) found no evidence of an antidepressant response but instead found significantly more side effects from the tricyclic-neuroleptic combination. In using antidepressant-neuroleptic combinations, a balance must be struck between the potential for therapeutic effect and the risk of incurring adverse or diminished antipsychotic effects.

COMMENT ON RESEARCH AND CLINICAL CARE

With increasing attention by newspapers and other media focused on advances in medical science, it is not uncommon to encounter a patient or family who knows of a "new" treatment and requests its use. Similarly, the clinician faced with the chronicity and severity of the schizophrenic illness in some patients may wish to turn to the latest research report holding the prospect of a better treatment for the patient. Although hope and tenacity in clinical care must never be abandoned, neither should sound management be replaced by a search for a cure that has yet to be found.

The task of discerning experimental work important for testing an etiologic hypothesis from that with direct clinical application often falls to the consultant. The administration of β-endorphin (Kline et al. 1977) or the use of hemodialysis (Wagemaker and

Cade 1977) are just two examples of what were touted at first as therapeutic breakthroughs for schizophrenia, only to later be shown to be ineffective in controlled studies (Pickar et al. 1981; Carpenter et al. 1983, respectively). It is hoped that in future years focused scientific research (or well-placed serendipity) will result in new drugs or procedures with a clinically meaningful impact on schizophrenia. Until then, judicious use of available pharmacotherapies in tandem with psychosocial supports and therapy represent the best approach for treating schizophrenia.

REFERENCES

Abrams R, Taylor MA: Catatonia: a prospective clinical study. Arch Gen Psychiatry 33:579–581, 1976

Abrams R, Taylor MA: A rating scale for emotional blunting. Am J Psychiatry 135:226–229, 1978

Alexander PE, Van Kammen DP, Bunney WE Jr: Antipsychotic effects of lithium in schizophrenia. Am J Psychiatry 136:283–287, 1979

American Psychiatric Association: Diagnostic and Statistical Manual of Mental Disorders (Third Edition). Washington, DC, American Psychiatric Association, 1980

Anderson WH, Kuehnle JD, Cantanzano DM: Rapid treatment of acute psychosis. Am J Psychiatry 133:1076–1078, 1976

Andreasen NC, Olsen SA, Denvert JW, et al: Ventricular enlargement in schizophrenia: relationship to positive and negative symptoms. Am J Psychiatry 139:297–306, 1982

Atsmon A, Blum I, Stewer M, et al: Further studies with propranolol in psychiatric patients. Psychopharmacologia 27:249–254, 1972

Ayd FJ: The depot fluphenazines: a reappraisal after 10 years' clinical experience. Am J Psychiatry 132:491–500, 1975

Bacher NM, Lewis HA: Addition of reserpine to antipsychotic medication in refractory chronic schizophrenic outpatients. Am J Psychiatry 135:488–489, 1978

Baldessarini RJ: Drugs and the treatment of psychiatric disorders, in The Pharmacologic Basis of Therapeutics. Edited by Gilman AG, Goodman LS, Gilman A. New York, Macmillan, 1980

Baldessarini RJ, Tarsy DT: Relationship of the actions of neuroleptic drugs to the pathophysiology of tardive dyskinesia. Int Rev Neurobiol 21:1–45, 1979

Baron M, Gruen R, Asnis L, et al: Schizoaffective illness, schizophrenia and affective disorders: morbidity risk and genetic transmission. Acta Psychiatr Scand 65:253–262, 1982

Barsa JA, Line NS: Combined reserpine–chlorpromazine in treatment of disturbed psychotics. Arch Neurol Psychiatry 74:280–286, 1955

Belmaker RH, Ebstein RP, Dasberg H, et al: The effect of propranolol treatment in schizophrenia on CSF amine metabolites and prolactin. Psychopharmacology 63:293–296, 1979

Berrios GE: Positive and negative symptoms and Jackson. Arch Gen Psychiatry 42:95–97, 1985

Birkhimer LJ, DeVane CL: The neuroleptic malignant syndrome: presentation and treatment. Drug Intell Clin Pharm 18:462–465, 1984

Bjorndal N, Bjerre M, Gerlach J, et al: High dosage haloperidol therapy in chronic schizophrenic patients. Psychopharmacology 67:17–23, 1980

Bowers MB, Astrachan BM: Depression in acute schizophrenic psychosis. Am J Psychiatry 123:976–981, 1967

Braun M: Reserpine as a therapeutic agent in schizophrenia. Am J Psychiatry 116:747, 1960

Bunney BS: Antipsychotic drug effects on the electrical activity of dopaminergic neurons. Trends in Neuroscience Research 7:212–215, 1984

Bunney BS, Grace AA: Acute and chronic haloperidol treatment: comparison of effects on nigral dopaminergic cell activity. Life Sci 23:1715–1728, 1978

Bunney BS, Walters JR, Roth RH, et al: Dopaminergic neurons: effect of antipsychotic drugs and amphetamine on single cell activity. J Pharmacol Exp Ther 185:560–571, 1973

Bunney WE Jr, Hamburg DA: Methods for reliable longitudinal observations of behavior. Arch Gen Psychiatry 9:280–294, 1963

Carlsson A: Antipsychotic drugs, neurotransmitters and schizophrenia. Am J Psychiatry 135:164–173, 1978

Carlsson A, Lindquist M: Effect of chlorpromazine or haloperidol on formation of 3-methoxytyramine and normetanephrine in mouse brain. Acta Pharmacol Toxicol 20:140, 1963

Caroff SN: The neuroleptic malignant syndrome. J Clin Psychiatry 41:79–82, 1980

Carpenter WT, Sadler JH, Light PD, et al: The therapeutic efficacy of hemodialysis in schizophrenia. N Engl J Med 308:669–675, 1983

Cohen WJ, Cohen NM: Lithium carbonate, haloperidol and irreversible brain damage. JAMA 230:1283–1287, 1974

Creese I, Burt DR, Snyder SH: Dopamine receptor binding predicts clinical and pharmacologic potencies of antischizophrenic drugs. Science 192:481–483, 1976

Crow TJ: Molecular pathology of schizophrenia: more than one disease process? Br Med J 280:66–68, 1980

Crow TJ: Positive and negative schizophrenia symptoms and the role of dopamine. Br J Psychiatry 139:251–254, 1981

Csernansky JG, Lombrozo L, Gulevich GD, et al: Treatment of negative schizophrenic symptoms with alprazolam: a preliminary open-label study. J Clin Psychopharmacol 4:349–351, 1984

Davis JM: Overview: maintenance therapy in psychiatry: I. Schizophrenia. Am J Psychiatry 133:1237–1245, 1975

Davis J, Janicak P, Linden R, et al: Neuroleptics and Psychotic Disorders, in Neuroleptics: Neurochemical, Behavioral and Clinical Perspectives. Edited by Coyle JT, Enna SJ. New York, Raven Press, 1983

Dawson GW, Jue SG, Brogden RN: Alprazolam: a review of its pharmacodynamic properties and efficacy in the treatment of anxiety and depression. Drugs 27:132–147, 1984

Delay J, Deniker P: Trente-huit cas de psychoses tratées par la cure prolongée et continue de 4560 RP. Le Congres des Al. et Neurol de Langue Fr. In Compte Rendu des Congrès, Masson et Cie, Paris, 1952

Delva NJ, Letemendia FJJ: Lithium treatment in schizophrenia and schizoaffective disorders. Br J Psychiatry 141:387–400, 1982

DeVogelaer J: Carbamazepine in the treatment of psychotic and behavioral disorders. Acta Psychiatr Belg 81:532–554, 1981

Docherty JP, van Kammen DP, Siris SG, et al: Stages of onset of schizophrenic psychosis. Am J Psychiatry 135:420–426, 1978

Donaldson SR, Gelenberg AS, Baldessarini RJ: The pharmacologic treatment of schizophrenia: a progress report. Schizophr Bull 9:504–527, 1983

Donlon PT: High dosage neuroleptic therapy: a review. International Journal of Pharmacopsychiatry 22:235–245, 1976

Donlon PT, Blacker KN: Stages of schizophrenia decompensation and reintegration. J Nerv Ment Dis 157:200–208, 1973

Donlon PT, Tupin JP: Rapid "digitalization" of decompensated schizophrenic patients with antipsychotic agents. Am J Psychiatry 132:1023–1026, 1975

Eissler KR: Remarks on the psycho-analysis of schizophrenia. Int J Psychoanal 32:139–156, 1951

Gardos C, Cole JO, Volicer L, et al: A dose response study of propranolol in chronic schizophrenics. Current Therapeutic Research 15:314–323, 1973

Gelenberg AJ, Mandel MR: Catatonic reactions to high-potency neuroleptic drugs. Arch Gen Psychiatry 34:947–950, 1977

Gershon ES, Hamovit J, Guroff JJ, et al: A family study of schizoaffective, bipolar I, bipolar II, unipolar, and normal control probands. Arch Gen Psychiatry 39:1157–1167, 1982

Goldberg SC, Frosch WA, Prossman AK, et al: Prediction of response to phenothiazines in schizophrenia: a cross validation study. Arch Gen Psychiatry 26:367–373, 1972

Growe GA, Clayton JW, Klass DB, et al: Lithium in chronic schizophrenia. Am J Psychiatry 136:454–455, 1979

Hakolu HPA, Laulumaa VAO: Carbamazepine in the treatment of violent schizophrenics. Lancet 1:1358, 1982

Henderson VW, Wosten GF: Neuroleptic malignant syndrome: a pathogenetic role for dopamine receptor blockade. Neurology 31:132–136, 1981

Hogarty GE, Goldberg SC, Schooler NE, et al: Drug and sociotherapy in the aftercare of schizophrenic patients. II: two year relapse rates. Arch Gen Psychiatry 31:603–608, 1975

Hogarty GE, Munetz MR: Pharmacogenic depression among outpatient schizophrenic patients: a failure to substantiate. J Clin Psychopharmacol 4:17–24, 1984

Hollister LF, Overall JE, Kimbell I, et al: Specific indications for different classes of phenothiazines. Arch Gen Psychiatry 30:94–99, 1974

Insel TR, Ninan PT, Aloi J, et al: A benzodiazepine receptor-mediated model of anxiety. Arch Gen Psychiatry 41:741–750, 1984

Iversen LL: Dopamine receptors in brain. Science 188:1084–1089, 1975

Jeste DV, Wyatt RJ: In search of treatment of tardive dyskinesia: review of the literature. Schizophr Bull 5:251–293, 1979

Johnson DAW: Studies of depressive symptoms in schizophrenia. I. The prevalence of depression and its possible causes. Br J Psychiatry 139:89–93, 1981a

Johnson DAW: Studies of depressive symptoms in schizophrenia. II. A two year longitudinal study of symptoms. Br J Psychiatry 139:93–96, 1981b

Johnson DAW: Studies of depressive symptoms in schizophrenia. IV. A double-blind trial of nortriptyline for depression in chronic schizophrenia. Br J Psychiatry 139:97–101, 1981c

Kebabian JW, Petzold GL, Greengard P: Dopamine-sensitive adenylate cyclase in candate nucleus of rat brain and its similarity to the "dopamine receptor." Proc Natl Acad Sci USA 79:2145–2149, 1972

Kendler KS: Paranoia (delusional disorder): a valid psychiatric entity? Trends in Neuroscience Research 7:14–17, 1984

Kety SS: The syndrome of schizophrenia: unresolved questions and opportunities for research. Br J Psychiatry 136:421–436, 1980

Klein E, Bental E, Lerer B, et al: Carbamazepine and haloperidol vs placebo and haloperidol in excited psychosis. Arch Gen Psychiatry 41:165–170, 1984

Kline NS, Li CH, Lehmann HE, et al: β-endorphin induced changes in schizophrenic and depressed patients. Arch Gen Psychiatry 34:1111–1113, 1977

Knights A, Okasha MS, Salitt MA, et al: Depressive and extraypyramidal symptoms and clinical effects: a trial of fluphenazine versus flupenthixol in maintenance of schizophrenic outpatients. Br J Psychiatry 135:515–523, 1979

Lerner P, Nose P, Cordon EK, et al: Haloperidol: effect of long-term treatment on rat striatal dopamine synthesis and turnover. Science 197:181–183, 1977

Lindstrom LH, Persson E: Propranolol in chronic schizophrenia: a controlled study in neuroleptic-treated patients. Br J Psychiatry 137:126–130, 1980

Lipinski JF, Zubenko GS, Cohen BM, et al: Propranolol in the treatment of neuroleptic-induced akathesia. Am J Psychiatry 141:412–415, 1984

Luchins DJ: Carbamazepine for the violent psychiatric patient. Lancet 2:766, 1983

Mandel MR, Severe JB, Schooler NR, et al: Development and prediction of postpsychotic depression in neuroleptic-treated schizophrenics. Arch Gen Psychiatry 39:197–203, 1982

Marder SR, Van Kammen DP, Docherty JP, et al: Predicting drug-free improvement in schizophrenic psychosis. Arch Gen Psychiatry 36:1080–1085, 1979

Mattes JA, Nayak D: Lithium versus fluphenazine for prophylaxis in mainly schizophrenic schizo-affectives. Biol Psychiatry 19:445–449, 1984

May DC, Morris SW, Stewart RM, et al: Neuroleptic malignant syndrome: response to dantrolen sodium. Ann Intern Med 98:183–184, 1983

Mayer-Gross W: Uber die Stellungsnahme auf abgelaufenen akuten Psychose. Zeitschrift für die Gesamte Neurol Psychiatr 60:160–212, 1920

McGlashan FH, Carpenter WT: Postpsychotic depression in schizophrenia. Arch Gen Psychiatry 33:231–239, 1976

Meltzer HY, Kane JM, Kalakowska T: Plasma levels of neuroleptics, prolactin and clinical response, in Neuroleptics: Neurochemical, Behavioral and Clinical Perspectives. Edited by Coyle JT, Enna SJ. New York, Raven Press, 1983

Meltzer HY, Stahl SM: The dopamine hypothesis of schizophrenia: a review. Schizophr Bull 2:19–76, 1976

Morrison JR: Changes in subtype diagnosis of schizophrenia, 1920–1966. Am J Psychiatry 131:674–677, 1974

Nasrallah HA, Donnelly EF, Bigelow LB, et al: Inhibition of dopamine synthesis in chronic schizophrenia. Arch Gen Psychiatry 34:649–655, 1977

Neborsky R, Janowsky D, Murson E, et al: Rapid treatment of acute psychotic symptoms with high and low-dose haloperidol. Arch Gen Psychiatry 38:195–199, 1981

Neppe VM: Carbamazepine in the psychiatric patient. Lancet 2:334, 1982

Overall JE, Gorham DE: The brief psychiatric rating scale. Psychol Rep 10:799–812, 1961

Peet M, Bethell MS, Coates A, et al: Propranolol in schizophrenia. I. Comparison of propranolol, chlorpromazine and placebo. Br J Psychiatry 139:105–111, 1981

Pickar D, Davis GC, Schulz SC, et al: Behavioral and biological effects of acute β-endorphin injection in schizophrenic and depressed patients. Am J Psychiatry 138:160–166, 1981

Pickar D, Labarca R, Linnoila M, et al: Neuroleptic-induced decrease in plasma homovanillic acid and antipsychotic activity in schizophrenic patients. Science 225:954–957, 1984

Pope HG, Lipinski JF, Cohen BM, et al: "Schizoaffective Disorder": an invalid diagnosis? A comparison of schizoaffective disorder, schizophrenia and affective disorder. Am J Psychiatry 137:921–927, 1980

Post RM: Use of the anticonvulsant carbamazepine in primary and secondary affective illness: clinical and theoretical implications (Editorial). Psychol Med 12:701–704, 1982

Post RM, Uhde TW, Ballenger JC, et al: Prophylactic efficacy of carbamazepine in manic–depressive illness. Am J Psychiatry 140:1602–1604, 1983

Prusoff BA, Williams DH, Weissman MM, et al: Treatment of secondary depression in schizophrenia. Arch Gen Psychiatry 36:569–575, 1979

Quitkin F, Rifkin A, Klein DF: Very high dosage vs standard dosage of fluphenazine in schizophrenia. Arch Gen Psychiatry 32:1276–1281, 1975

Richelson E: Neuroleptic affinities for human brain receptors and their use in predicting adverse effects. J Clin Psychiatry 45:331–336, 1984

Rorn S: The seemingly ubiquitous depression following acute schizophrenic episodes: a neglected area of clinical discussion. Am J Psychiatry 127:51–58, 1970

Roth RH: Neuroleptics: functional neurochemistry, in Neuroleptics: Neurochemical, Behavioral and Clinical Perspectives. Edited by Coyle JT, Enna SJ. New York, Raven Press, 1983

Roth RH, Bacopoulos NG, Bustos G, et al: Antipsychotic drugs: differential effects on dopamine neurons in basal ganglia and meso-cortex following chronic administration in human and nonhuman primates. Adv Biochem Psychopharmacol 24:513–520, 1980

Roy A: Depression in the course of chronic undifferentiated schizophrenia. Arch Gen Psychiatry 38:296–300, 1981

Roy A, Mazonson A, Pickar D: Attempted suicide in chronic schizophrenia. Br J Psychiatry 144:303–306, 1984

Seeman P, Lee T, Chau-Wong M, et al: Brain receptors for antipsychotic drug doses and neuroleptic/dopamine receptors. Nature 261:717–719, 1976

Shopsin B, Kim SS, Gershon S: A controlled study of lithium vs chlorpromazine in acute schizophrenics. Br J Psychiatry 119:435–440, 1971

Siris SG, Van Kammen DP, Docherty JP: Use of antidepressant drugs in schizophrenia. Arch Gen Psychiatry 35:1368–1377, 1978

Skolnick P, Paul SM: Benzodiazepine receptors in the central nervous system. Int Rev Neurobiol 23:103–140, 1982

Small JG, Kellams JJ, Milstein V, et al: A placebo controlled study of lithium combined with neuroleptics in chronic schizophrenia. Am J Psychiatry 132:1315–1317, 1975

Spitzer RL, Endicott JE, Robins E: Research diagnostic criteria (RDC) for a selected group of functional disorders. New York State Psychiatric Institute, Biometrics Research Unit, 1975

Stevens JR: An anatomy of schizophrenia. Arch Gen Psychiatry 29:177–189, 1973

Stevens JR, Bigelow L, Denney D, et al: Telemetered EEG–EOG during psychotic behaviors of schizophrenia. Arch Gen Psychiatry 36:251–269, 1979

Stoudemire A: The differential diagnosis of catatonic states. Psychosomatics 23:245–251, 1982

Strauss JS, Gift TE: Choosing an approach for diagnosing schizophrenia. Arch Gen Psychiatry 34:1248–1253, 1977

Strauss JS, Carpenter WT: Schizophrenia. New York, Plenum Press, 1982

Tamminga CA, Schaffer MH, Smitlo RC, et al: Apomorphine improves schizophrenic symptoms. Science 200:567–568, 1978

Taylor MA, Abrams R: Catatonia: prevalence and importance in the manic phase of manic–depressive illness. Arch Gen Psychiatry 34:1223–1225, 1977

Tsuang MT: "Schizoaffective Disorder": dead or alive? Arch Gen Psychiatry 36:633–634, 1979

Van Kammen DP, Alexander PE, Bunney WE Jr: Lithium treatment in postpsychotic depression. Br J Psychiatry 136:479–485, 1980

Wagemaker H, Cade R: The use of hemodialysis in chronic schizophrenia. Am J Psychiatry 134:684–685, 1977

Weinberger DR: Brain disease and psychiatric illness: when should a psychiatrist order a CAT scan? Am J Psychiatry 141:1521–1532, 1984

Weinberger DR, Bigelow LB, Kleinman JE, et al: Cerebral ventricular enlargement in chronic schizophrenia. Arch Gen Psychiatry 37:11–13, 1980

White FJ, Wang RY: Differential effects of classical and atypical antipsychotic drugs on A_9 and A_{10} dopamine neurons. Science 221:1054–1056, 1983

Willander J, Skott A, Carlsson A, et al: Potentiation by metyrosine of thioridazine effects in chronic schizophrenics. Arch Gen Psychiatry 33:501–505, 1976

Yorkston NJ, Zaki SA, Molek MKU, et al: Propranolol in the control of schizophrenic symptoms. Br Med J 10:633–635, 1974

Yorkston NJ, Pitcher DR, Gruzelier JH, et al: Propranolol as an adjunct to the treatment of schizophrenia. Lancet 2:575–578, 1977

Zarifian E, Scatton B, Bianchetti G, et al: High doses of haloperidol in schizophrenia. Arch Gen Psychiatry 39:212–215, 1982

Zemlam FP, Hirschowitz J, Santler FJ, et al: Impact of lithium therapy on core psychotic symptoms of schizophrenia. Br J Psychiatry 144:64–69, 1984

5

Clinical Psychopharmacology Consultation in the General Hospital

Edward L. Scharfman, M.D.

5

Clinical Psychopharmacology Consultation in the General Hospital

Psychiatrists have for some time been consultants for their colleagues on inpatients from medical, surgical, neurological, and gynecological services. Often the patients are management problems in that they evoke negative reactions from staff by being uncooperative, hostile, or noncompliant with work-ups, diet and rest restrictions, or medication. At other times consultations are requested for patients with chronic pain, psychophysiological disorders, overdoses, conversion, adverse drug reactions, and the ubiquitous "altered mental status." Of course, consultations are also requested on patients with a psychiatric history or those already on psychotropics who have concurrent medical or surgical problems.

The rapidly expanding frontier of new medications in general, and of psychotropic medications in particular, has created the demand for a psychiatric consultant with more subspecialized skills and expertise, that is, the clinical psychopharmacologist. The name itself captures the truly hybrid nature of this subspecialty. As a clinician, the psychiatric consultant needs to have a thorough background not only in psychopathology but in medicine and neurology as well, as so many medical and neurological

I wish to thank Richard I. Shader, M.D., for reviewing this manuscript and for his helpful suggestions and comments.

disorders and the medications used to treat them can mimic, aggravate, and even present as psychiatric disorders. As a clinical pharmacologist, the psychiatric consultant needs to be well versed in pharmacokinetics and drug–drug interactions not only of psychotropics, but of nonpsychotropic medications. Finally, as a psychiatrist, the psychiatric consultant needs the skills to understand, recognize, and work with "psychokinetics" and "people–people" interactions. I use these terms to connote the dynamic, latent forces of interactional processes intrinsic to the primary-physician (or nonphysician therapist)–consultant relationship, the primary-physician–patient relationship, and the consultant–patient relationship. Clinical pharmacologists have little experience in psychokinetics and people–people interactions, and clinical consultant-liaison psychiatrists, even when well versed in the use of psychotropics, often do not have expertise in pharmacokinetics and drug–drug interactions, especially of nonpsychotropic medications. The raison d'être of the consulting clinical psychopharmacologist is his or her ability to combine this variety of skills and expertise as clinician, consultant-liaison psychiatrist, and clinical pharmacologist and apply them to the consultation setting.

The hybrid nature of this subspecialty is illustrated with clinical vignettes from my experience consulting to nonpsychiatric physicians, psychiatrists, and nonphysician psychotherapists.

Working as a member of a psychiatric-liaison consultation team on call to the general hospital, I selectively fielded those consultations addressed to "psychopharmacology." Most often the patients requiring evaluation had primary medical, surgical, neurological, or gynecological illnesses and developed psychiatric symptoms secondary to the underlying illness or to medications used to treat that illness. (Issues concerning consultation to psychiatrists and nonphysician psychotherapists are discussed later in the chapter.)

As psychiatrists, we more than our colleagues in other medical specialties, should be sensitive to several factors before the consultation is initiated. The consultant must read between the lines and go straight to the latent content of the consultation request in order to understand the following points: a) What is the primary physician asking for; what does he or she want to hear? b) Perhaps even more important, what does the primary physician *not* want to hear? c) How can the consultant make the necessary recommendations in such a way as to have them carried out?

These principles are obviously not unique to psychopharmacological consultation, but the astute clinical psychopharmacologist, because he or she is trained in psychokinetics and people–people interactions, should be effective in having his or her suggestions carried out.

A primary physician requesting a consultation has several concerns and fears. First, there is the realization that he or she is stuck and needs help with a difficult case. This, in and of itself, is a potential narcissistic injury stirring up such feelings as failure, helplessness, and impotence. Second, the primary physician wonders whether he or she has missed something obvious or has been careless, negligent, or less than thorough. Third, the primary physician wonders whether the consulting specialist will provide recommendations from within the primary physician's specialty field, thus implying that he or she *has* missed something obvious.

These concerns are even more intense when the consultant is not seen as a "real doctor" by the primary physician, an unfortunate but prevalent attitude still held about psychiatrists by many nonpsychiatric physicians.

CLINICAL CASES

The clinical vignettes that follow are presented precisely the way the consultation form appeared in my mailbox. Just as psychiatrists begin forming impressions of prospective patients during the initial phone contact *before* the first session, so too must the consulting clinical psychopharmacologist begin to form impressions of the primary physician, the patient, and the milieu in which they are operating, by paying close attention to the wording and the tone of the consultation request.

Case 1

TO: PSYCHOPHARMACOLOGY

FROM: GASTROENTEROLOGY

How much haloperidol can safely be given to a 54-year-old woman with hepatitis and schizophrenia who has elevated liver function tests?

By the wording of this consultation the psychiatrist quickly understands what the primary physician wants to hear and what he or she does not want to hear. Not only has a psychiatric diagnosis been made, the neuroleptic to be used has already been chosen. The consultant is "reminded" that haloperidol is metabolized by the liver, and hepatitis is a disease that compromises liver function. Psychiatric skills will be as crucial as pharmacological skills for such a consultation to be effective. Nevertheless, the team is asking for help, and the patient is probably in trouble. On interview, the patient was jaundiced with ascites, and behaved in a guarded, suspicious, hypervigilant manner. She had recently been moved to a private room furthest from the nursing station, after accusing both the nursing staff and her previous roommates of plotting against her. She asked whether the consultant saw the three dead bodies of her visitors outside in the car on the street, and made references to special communications she received from the hospital page system. The family reported the acute onset of these symptoms during the preceding three days, and reported similar behavior three and one-half years earlier, "the first time mother's liver acted up." There was no other premorbid psychiatric history, and no family psychiatric history. She had been working as a bookkeeper for 13 years in the same firm up until admission to the gastroenterology (GI) service seven days earlier. She had been happily married for 29 years. Neurological exam by the consultant revealed first-degree horizontal nystagmus, bilateral resting hand tremor, and asterixis, findings that were not noted in the patient's record.

The diagnosis of hepatic encephalopathy with psychosis was no great feat, and the recommendations were geared at treating the underlying illness with a protein-restricted diet, lactulose, neomycin, and monitoring of serum ammonia levels and EEGs if desired. The difficulty was communicating this to the consultors without offending or threatening them. The house staff was actually quite receptive to a talk about differentiating organic and functional psychoses and diagnostic criteria for schizophrenia. The reproducible neurological findings impressed on them that the consultant was a "real doctor."

The attending was not so receptive, however, insisting, as a subspecialist himself, that patients with hepatic encephalopathy do not have visual hallucinations. Why could the consultant not simply provide guidelines for the use of the haloperidol? That is what the consultor wanted to hear. Having made an alliance with the house staff, an attempt was made to reach the attending through them. An article by the noted British hepatologist, Sheila Sherlock, on the neuropsychiatric manifestations of hepatic encephalopathy (Summerskill et al. 1956) was distributed, with her references to patients with visual hallucinations underlined, and it was suggested that it may be easier for the attending to receive this article from them, rather than from the consultant. Not only were the recommendations followed, but the patient's psychiatric symptoms remitted, and the very same GI team reconsulted on another case the next week.

Case 2

TO: PSYCHOPHARMACOLOGY

FROM: GASTROENTEROLOGY

31-year-old man, peptic ulcer disease, on imipramine started by private psychiatrist months prior to admission; appears toxic despite no change in dose. Please make recommendations.

Note the contrast in the wording of this request received from the same GI team, compared with the previous consultation. This one is less restrictive, giving the consultant a free license to "make recommendations." An alliance between consultors and consultant had been formed.

Major depression with melancholia was confirmed by the patient's psychiatrist, and the patient had just begun to respond to imipramine 200 mg/day. However, after a diagnosis of peptic ulcer disease was made, the patient was begun on cimetidine 300 mg q.i.d. 10 days earlier, on admission to the GI service. The patient was now experiencing severe dry mouth, constipation, flushing, and tachycardia without evidence of blood loss or hypovolemia. Cimetidine is known to produce a drug–drug interaction in which imipramine blood levels can be increased two- to threefold after the addition of cimetidine (Henauer and Hollister 1984). A trough imipramine level revealed an imipramine plus desipramine level of 415 ng, twice the minimum therapeutic blood level. Two recommendations were made: (a) decrease the imipramine for as long as the patient required cimetidine, and (b) consider switching to the H_2 blocker ranitidine, which in preliminary reports did not cause this interaction with imipramine (Abernethy et al. 1984). Only the first was followed, but the GI team was grateful to learn about the interaction of cimetidine and imipramine and that this did not occur with ranitidine.

Case 3

TO: PSYCHOPHARMACOLOGY

FROM: GENERAL SURGERY

44-year-old woman, pancreatitis, N.P.O., nasogastric suction, extremely anxious. Please advise on the use of parenteral anxiolytics.

The surgical team was aware of the pharmacokinetic property that benzodiazepines are erratically absorbed when administered intramuscularly. They were too concerned about respiratory depression to administer them intravenously. An earlier trial of intramuscular barbiturate caused oversedation and sleep, an effect neither the patient nor the team wanted. A trial of sublingual lorazepam was suggested, after an explanation that trans-mucous membrane absorption of lorazepam produces quick, reliable blood levels (Greenblatt et al. 1982). Such information was of great value to the surgical staff, who frequently have anxious patients who are also n.p.o. The recommendation was followed with good results of anxiolysis without sedation.

Case 4

TO: PSYCHOPHARMACOLOGY

FROM: CARDIOLOGY

71-year-old man, 4 weeks post MI, first degree A–V block, depressed, withdrawn, not participating in rehab. . . . Please advise. . . . Are antidepressants indicated? . . . Are they safe?

A thorough discussion of the literature on this topic with the cardiology team, stressing the safety of heterocyclics in such patients given close monitoring with telemetry still left them uneasy. The patient was losing weight, refusing visitors, and refusing to get out of bed. His history revealed a depressive episode 40 years earlier with an inability to go to work. The team agreed that in this case depression carried an increased risk of morbidity and mortality. Based on studies demonstrating the antidepressant properties of alprazolam at dosages of about 4 mg/day (Feighner et al. 1983), and given its low cardiotoxic profile, a trial with it was begun in addition to behavioral and supportive therapy. The cardiology team was greatly relieved to find an alternative to the heterocyclics in such a patient. The patient had a noticeable response within 11 days.

Case 5

TO: PSYCHOPHARMACOLOGY

FROM: INFECTIOUS DISEASE

> 28-year-old gay man, acquired immune deficiency syndrome, not eating, withdrawn, losing weight, giving up. . . . Please advise on usefulness of psychostimulants, anti-depressants.

The patient was terminal yet highly invested in by the staff, who had done everything possible during his seven-week hospitalization. They had tried every procedure, diagnostic test, drug, and consultation, all in vain. Cachectic and stuporous in his reverse isolation room, he could not even participate in an interview with the consultant. All members of the team conceded that he had one to two weeks to live; but if only he would eat or drink; maybe a magic bullet from the psychopharmacologist? Their request for a psychostimulant for the patient was based on their knowledge that tricyclic antidepressants take 10–14 days to work and that he would probably be dead by then. Would amphetamine or methylphenidate work where the experimental antibiotic AZ 1234 had failed?
It was the staff who needed the antidepressant and it was toward their collective feelings of defeat, failure, helplessness, and rage that the consultation efforts were directed. The consultant joined them by admitting that there were no magic bullets but allowed them to ventilate their sadness and frustration, and was empathic and supportive. The patient died four days later. About a month later the staff told the consultant that they were better able to integrate the experience of the patient's death having had the "T-group meeting."

Case 6

TO: PSYCHOPHARMACOLOGY

FROM: HEMATOLOGY/ONCOLOGY

> 32-year-old woman with acute lymphocytic leukemia on chemo regimen; possibly delusional about CNS metastases; lumbar punc-

ture and CT Scan are negative; Agitated; please evaluate and make recommendations.

The patient had been "agitated" ever since her neck became stiff, her tongue became heavy, and her arms started "jerking." This had never happened before her admission and was causing her great distress. She wondered whether the cancer was spreading to her spinal cord. She showed no evidence of delusional thinking or psychosis. A review of her medications revealed that she was on metoclopromide for chemotherapy-induced nausea. A talk with the staff on the recognition and treatment of dystonias induced by dopamine blockers was well received. Most of them did not even know that metoclopromide is a phenothiazine, and all remarked on how it was "used here like water." The patient responded rapidly to intravenous diphenhydramine with immediate relief of her "agitation."

These vignettes were chosen specifically to highlight the heterogeneous nature of cases the clinical consulting psychopharmacologist is likely to face in a general hospital. Obviously, such a hybrid subspecialist must have the combined skills and expertise of clinician, psychiatrist, and pharmacologist.

Consultation to other psychiatrists and nonphysician psychotherapists differs from consultation to nonpsychiatric physicians. The setting from which my experience is derived is the outpatient psychiatry and psychopharmacology clinic, and the inpatient psychiatry unit of the general hospital.

Contrary to the attitude of nonpsychiatric physicians, the psychopharmacologist is seen by his or her mental health colleagues as the expert, the "real doctor." In addition, because the clinical psychopharmacologist is a mental health professional, the stage is set for competition, resentment, and splitting. Moreover, when medications are recommended, the primary psychotherapist may need help in combining psychotherapy and pharmacotherapy.

The clinical psychopharmacologist is frequently asked to evaluate patients who are "stuck" in psychotherapy, who are diagnostic dilemmas, or "treatment failures." Often these patients have diagnoses in a grey area, such as subsyndromal affective disorders like cyclothymia and dysthymia, atypical depression, rejection-sensitive dysphoria, residual attention deficit disorder, emotionally unstable character disorder, and schizotypal disorder. The expectation is that the psychopharmacologist has the magic bullet to palliate if not cure them. This puts an enormous burden on the consultant to *act*, that is, to *prescribe*. However, one hallmark of a good psychopharmacologist is knowing when not to prescribe, and recognizing when the pressure to prescribe is coming from the consultor for his or her own sake more than for the patient's sake. On the other hand, several patients with these diagnoses are otherwise labeled as "borderline," and many may in fact benefit from pharmacotherapy.

A most unfortunate, seemingly paradoxical, but not uncommon experience is the primary psychotherapist who covertly hopes that the psychopharmacologist will fail. This phenomenon is not restricted to nonphysician psychotherapists, but is common among all psychotherapists who share a reductionistic, simplistic view of psychopathology rather than a multidimensional biopsychosocial one. Often the underlying fear is that a beneficial pharmacological response by their patients would in some way invalidate and devalue their theory of psychopathology and their practice of psychotherapy.

Splitting is often encountered when the patient values the "pills" and devalues the "talking therapy." The patient may prefer to use his or her outpatient insurance for the psychopharmacology meetings, and begins to miss or cancel the psychotherapy sessions. Such cases require a close partnership between the primary psychotherapist and the consultant to prevent the possible acting-out of the patient's pathology, and to present a consistent therapeutic front to the patient by both psychotherapist and psychopharmacologist. A discussion between the psychopharmacologist and the patient of the realistic expectations for the medication and the adjunct role it serves can often prevent magic overidealization of the psychopharmacologist and devaluation of the psychotherapist.

A most fascinating phenomenon is the development of intense transference to the psychopharmacologist that frequently unfolds even in patients who are seen only for half an hour once a month. The medication is not only a transitional object, it is an introject as well. Just as an interpretation is a part of the psychotherapist, so the medication is a part of the psychopharmacologist that is taken in by the patient, incorporated, and that then exerts effects on the patient's mind and body, effects that at times are beneficial, and at times toxic. Compliance with, response or lack of response to, and side effects from medication are all influenced to some degree by transference phenomena. The psychopharmacologist's failure to recognize and effectively deal with such transference phenomena could lead to treatment failure exactly the way failure to recognize and effectively deal with transference phenomena in psychotherapy could result in a negative therapeutic outcome.

These issues once again highlight the hybrid nature of this subspecialist. Abdicating the role of psychiatrist, and/or forgetting one's training in psychokinetics and people–people interactions would clearly impair the ability of the clinical psychopharmacologist to effectively and successfully contribute to the pharmacological field.

PERSPECTIVES ON CLINICAL TRAINING

Finally, a few thoughts about training the clinical psychopharmacologist. Training should be incorporated into the early years of residency programs to prevent the formation of narrowminded, inflexible attitudes by beginning residents. Too often one hears from postgraduate year 1 and 2 trainees that "this is a pure psychotherapy case" or "psychotherapy and pharmacotherapy have to be done by separate clinicians." Seminars, case conferences, and direct clinical experience should be geared to exposing trainees early on to conceptualizing psychopathology and formulating treatment plans according to a broad, multidimensional biopsychosocial model.

A clinical fellow should be immersed in working up and treating a wide variety of inpatients and outpatients, while working with consultors who are psychiatrists, nonphysician psychotherapists, and nonpsychiatric physicians. He or she should have regular access to supervision by one or more senior clinical psychopharmacologists, and have opportunities to observe his or her mentors in seminars and case conferences. Regular group supervision, in which unusual and atypical clinical cases are presented to and discussed by senior psychopharmacologists, provides fellows with fine-tuning and polish in their training that is unavailable in textbooks or journals. The fellow should be expected to teach students and residents in both didactic and clinical settings. He or she should be expected to participate in, or even design, a clinical study. Finally, a fellow should be encouraged to publish and present papers of interest and importance at seminars, conferences, grand rounds, and conventions.

REFERENCES

Abernethy DR, Greenblatt DJ, Eshelman FN, et al: Ranitidine does not impair oxidative or conjugative metabolism: noninteraction with antipyrine, diazepam and lorazepam. Clin Pharmacol Ther 35:188–192, 1984

Feighner JD, Aden GC, Fabre LF, et al: Comparison of alprazolam, imipramine, and placebo in the treatment of depression. JAMA 249:3057–3064, 1983

Glickman LS: Psychiatric Consultation in the General Hospital. New York, Marcel Decker, 1980

Greenblatt DJ, Divoll M, Harmatz JS, et al: Pharmacokinetic comparison of sublingual lorazepam with intravenous, intramuscular and oral lorazepam. J Pharmaceutical Sci 71:248–252, 1982

Henauer SA, Hollister LE: Cimetidine interaction with imipramine and nortriptyline. Clin Pharmacol Ther 35:183–187, 1984

Summerskill WHJ, Davidson EA, Sherlock S, et al: The neuropsychiatric syndrome associated with hepatic cirrhosis and an extensive portal collateral circulation. Q J Med 49:245–266, 1956

6

Psychopharmacology Evaluation: Psychosocial Issues

John P. Docherty, M.D.

6

Psychopharmacology Evaluation: Psychosocial Issues

The experienced practitioner is well aware that expert psychopharmacological treatment is not simply a matter of prescribing the right drug or combination of drugs for a particular disorder. Sophisticated and optimal treatment also entails careful attention to those psychosocial variables that may affect the ultimate outcome of the drug treatment regimen. For the practical purposes of this monograph, I have categorized these variables into three major groups and selected those items of pragmatic relevance to psychopharmacological therapy. The three categories are a) potential barriers to compliance with the prescribed regimen, b) special issues in psychotherapy that bear on the effectiveness of concomitant drug treatment, and c) psychosocial forces that inhibit or facilitate drug response.

COMPLIANCE: "THE SOUND OF ONE HAND CLAPPING"

A potentially effective treatment not used, or used inappropriately, will not be effective. Unfortunately, the rate of noncompliance with psychopharmacological treatments is extremely high, ranging from 30 to 60 percent depending on the type of disorder being treated and the duration of therapy (Blackwell 1979; Stimson 1974).

The Appendix to this chapter contains a checklist that the clinician may use to insure that basic questions bearing on compliance have been considered in a patient's treatment. The checklist consists of five categories. Each of these categories is discussed in turn.

The first category refers to the diagnosis of the presence and specific form of noncompliance (Section 1 of the Appendix). The exact nature of the noncompliance should be determined because it will dictate different forms of intervention. As the questions in the Appendix indicate, noncompliance can involve too much medication, too little medication, or the erratic and improper use of the medication. Furthermore, the way in which a person will take either too much or too little medication may differ. One individual may miss sporadic doses, another may miss days at a time, yet at the end of a week each may have taken the same amount of medication (Malahy 1966).

Finally, many studies have demonstrated that a physician's estimate based on "clinical intuition" is a very poor judgment of the degree of compliance (Gordis 1979). It is important, especially if the question of noncompliance arises, that other methods be used to determine the presence, degree, and form of noncompliance. These methods may entail supervision, observation by relatives, requesting that a patient bring in a pill bottle for a pill count, or the use of a structured interview that carefully and systematically examines the patient's pill taking behavior over a specified period.

If noncompliance seems to be present, the physician should then systematically examine the situation for those variables that may be contributing to the noncompliance. The first of these has to do with the patient him- or herself (Section 2 of the Appendix).

One initial question that the patient should be asked is the reason for his or her noncompliance. VanPutten (1978) has provided five helpful heuristic categories of commonly expressed or observed motives for noncompliance. These categories are useful because they suggest appropriate responses. The first is intelligent noncompliance, in which the patient changes the medication dosage because of uncomfortable or potentially dangerous side effects, yet does well on the new regimen. The second is capricious noncompliance, in which the patient, for no apparent reason, changes medication irregularly from day to day. The third is deliberate drug refusal, in which, for a variety of reasons, the patient simply objects to taking the medication. The fourth is confused compliance, in which the patient, because of disturbances in thinking and organizational competencies, is unable to follow the prescribed regimen. The fifth is misdirection noncompliance, an iatrogenic noncompliance, in which the patient, because of inadequate, incomplete, or improper directions, is not taking the medication in the appropriate fashion.

The next step involves the importance of taking a history of compliance behavior in individual patients. Although much noncompliance may be situationally induced and thus may come and go in individual patients, it is still more likely that patients with a past history of noncompliance will demonstrate that same behavior with a new medication.

The third focus addresses the important findings in the literature with regard to Rosenstock's "health belief" model (Becker and Maimen 1980). This model is a strong predictor of compliance behavior. It asserts that the likelihood that a patient will take medication as prescribed is strongly dependent on the patient's perception of the severity of the illness, of the likelihood of recurrence or worsening if the medication is stopped, the belief that the treatment will be helpful in alleviating the illness, and the perceived cost of the treatment in social, financial, psychological, or physical terms.

Fourth, it has been demonstrated that particular aspects of psychiatric disorders may affect compliance. This does not imply that such problems are not present in other medical patients. It refers, rather, to specific psychological phenomena that may undermine compliance. These include the patient's denial that an illness exists; cognitive disorganization, either through such illnesses as schizophrenia or dementia, that impair the person's ability to follow a treatment schedule; the presence of avoidance behavior as a characteristic coping mechanism that leads a patient to stay away from signifiers of the illness, such as the treatment itself; and irrational beliefs, primarily paranoidal and delusional concerns about the effect on treatment (Evans and Spelman 1983).

Fifth, it is important to examine the patient's current familial and social situation. Patients living in unstable social situations are more likely to evidence noncompliance. Moreover, negative attitudes on the part of family members toward the treatment may also lead to noncompliance. It is important for the physician to know whether such attitudes exist so they may be counteracted directly (Blackwell 1979; Stimson 1974).

The second major category of influence on the compliance of the patient has to do with the psychopharmacological regimen itself (Section 3 of the Appendix). The range of physiological effects of the medication raises two issues of concern: the compatibility for the patient of certain associated properties of the medication and the patient's tolerance of the medication's side effects.

In the checklist, sedation is singled out because for some patients and conditions it is desirable as an associate property and will enhance compliance, whereas for others it will diminish compliance. It is important that the clinician be aware of this. For some patients a cognitive dulling is a sought-after experience; for others it produces extreme dysphoria (Christensen 1978).

Secondly, the dosage schedule must be considered. Overall, the more complex the dosage schedule, the less compliance will be achieved. This includes variables such as the frequency of medication, dosage, variation in dosages, and variability of administration times. Additionally, the longer a medication is prescribed, the more likely it is that compliance problems will emerge (Becker and Maiman 1980).

Thirdly, the clinician must consider the degree of change required in the patient's daily routine in order to accommodate the drug treatment. To the extent that any change in the patient's routine can be minimized, compliance is more likely. As a result, associating dosing with regular mealtimes is an advantageous way to insure compliance. Any major need for change in the patient's daily schedule, however, may be an important source of noncompliance and should be specifically identified (Marston 1970).

Fourth, the route of administration must be considered. In

general, self-administered oral pills produce the least compliance. The obvious usefulness of switching to a liquid or a parenteral form of administration in appropriate situations should not be overlooked (Haynes 1976).

Finally, cost can be a consideration in noncompliance and should be taken into account. This is an issue that a patient is unlikely to bring up unless the doctor asks. The high cost of medication, especially for some patients whose therapy, but not drug treatment, is reimbursed through a third-party source, must be considered (Blackwell 1979).

A third major influence on a patient's compliance with a drug treatment derives from the relationship between the physician and the patient (Section 4 of the Appendix). Here several questions must be asked:

1. How explicit has the physician been in making clear exactly what the patient must do in order to carry out the treatment regimen?
2. Have the patient and doctor taken the time to discuss what their mutual expectations are for the treatment?
3. Has the patient clearly understood and acknowledged the necessary steps he or she must take in order to carry out the treatment program?
4. Finally, but extremely importantly, have the patient and doctor developed a positive and supportive tone in the relationship? As I discuss later in the chapter, both compliance behavior and the overall outcome of the treatment are enhanced if the tone of the relationship is maintained in this fashion (Docherty and Fiester 1985).

The last category of influence on compliance considered in the checklist is the overall treatment program setting (Section 5 in the Appendix). Several factors in this domain influence compliance. These include the continuity of care the patient is experiencing, both as regards the clinician taking care of him or her and the actual setting in which the treatment takes place, as well as such mundane issues as having a constant appointment time. Interruptions in any or all of these areas tend to decrease compliance. In essence, the main finding reported from this work is that the greater the regularity and stability of a patient's treatment program, the more likely compliance with the treatment program will be achieved (Ettlinger and Freedman 1981).

Intervention

Overall, it is important that the source of the noncompliance be carefully diagnosed and that an intervention be tailored to the particular problem causing the noncompliance. In general, however, the following suggestions may be kept in mind in order to prevent noncompliance from developing.

1. The treatment program should be made as clear and simple as possible. This may include giving the patient written instructions about using the medication, as well as providing a rationale for using the medication that is relevant to the patient's concerns.
2. The therapeutic program should be kept as simple as possible. This includes decreasing the daily dosage frequency to a minimum, incorporating taking the medication into the patient's daily routine, and using long-acting drugs whenever possible.
3. Side effects should be prevented or carefully minimized as they arise.
4. Any indications of beginning noncompliance should be met with increased monitoring, through specific questioning, the use of relative observation, pill counts, and so on.
5. The family should be informed either through the patient or directly about the nature of the patient's illness, the rationale for the use of the medication, as well as the specific drug treatment program undertaken. Similarly, side effects should be discussed in order to minimize the possibility that anxiety or concern over emerging side effects will lead to the discontinuation of the medication.
6. Finally, it is extremely important that the doctor–patient relationship receive careful attention.

PSYCHOTHERAPY AND PSYCHOPHARMACOLOGICAL TREATMENT

Psychotherapy research to date has found that the therapeutic alliance is the single most powerful variable in predicting psychotherapy outcome. This is true across a variety of different forms of psychotherapy (Hartley 1985). Pharmacotherapeutic treatment has demonstrated similarly that the doctor's attention to the doctor–patient interaction will strongly influence the outcome of the drug treatment program. This "warming up of the treatment" includes, but is not limited to, simply enhancing compliance with pharmacological treatment. It, at least, includes the enhancement of the associated placebo effects of the medication, and the so-called nonspecific psychological variables associated with recovery, such as the development of a feeling of hope, a sense of trust and confidence in a therapist, a feeling of safety and security in the therapeutic setting, and a sense that oneself and one's illness are understood by the therapist.

Based on a review of the medical compliance and psychotherapeutic alliance literature, the following type of overall doctor–patient relationship should result in an optimal degree of compliance. The relationship should involve a reciprocity of roles, with the patient feeling a sense of control and being involved as an active participant, and with the doctor actively sharing information, encouraging discussion of issues and providing feedback. It should be a relationship in which mutuality of expectations is achieved through a process of sharing both parties' expectations about treatment goals and the mechanisms of achieving these goals, and in which negotiation and collaborative decisionmaking take place. This should be a relationship in which the rights and responsibilities of both parties are clear; in which an optimal quantity of information is available in a comprehensive form on which decisions can be based (especially information about the treatment regimen). It should be a relationship in which a therapeutic environment is created where the patient experiences the doctor as warm, friendly, sympathetic, interested, respectful, concerned, and generally positive and supportive, not authoritarian, dominant, dogmatic, critical, or distant. In this type of relationship the patient is motivated and has a positive attitude; the patient's individual needs, abilities, and life circumstances are actively considered in the general therapeutic process; and there is active inquiry about and adequate attention given to the patient's perception of all these factors, particularly the patient's perception of the therapeutic relationship. Finally, it should be a relationship in which special attention is given to these factors in the critical early visits when it is first being established.

However, in conducting a combined treatment with drugs and psychotherapy, several other issues of which the doctor should be cognizant may interfere with the development of a positive feeling between the patient and physician (Docherty 1979). A listing of these issues follows.

1. The symbolic meaning of the medication—The medication may possess for the patient an untoward meaning that can negatively influence the patient's participation in the treatment or response to the therapist. If, for example, the patient sees the medication as an indicator that the therapist feels the patient is a bad person or incompetent to successfully complete a psychotherapeutic treatment, then the outcome will be negatively influenced. The therapist should inquire about the meaning of the medication for the patient and deal with any negative perceptions that are disclosed.
2. The problem of interpersonal continuity—A strong effect of the medication can radically change the nature of the ongoing doctor–patient relationship. For example, a withdrawn patient who begins to recover and goes through a period of increased energy, while still maintaining a depressive irritability, will behave in a very different fashion toward the physician—and without any significant relationship precipitant of this change. The physician should be aware of the biochemical process of change in the patient so that the relationship's continuity is not disturbed.
3. A substitute for discussing interpersonal difficulties—It can happen that medication is prescribed in order to deal with a

problem in the patient–therapist relationship. For example, if the patient is complaining that the therapist is not doing enough for him or her, the physician may respond by prescribing more medication. This may or may not be appropriate. It may be that in that particular situation the patient's needs and expectations must be discussed and modified, or that the physician should provide more help in some other way.

All in all, it is essential that the physician consider these issues in order to minimize their adverse effects on the effective implementation of a concomitant psychopharmacological treatment program.

OTHER PSYCHOSOCIAL INFLUENCES ON PHARMACOLOGICAL TREATMENT RESPONSE

This discussion has been limited to two issues that must be considered by the physician in conducting pharmacotherapy. The first is the affective nature of the social context. Important recent findings in the investigation of the maintenance treatment of schizophrenic patients show that the emotional climate in which the patient exists may strongly influence his or her response to a drug treatment program. It has been demonstrated that the presence of a high degree of hostility and criticism from those people with whom the schizophrenic patient lives and has frequent contact predisposes the patient to relapse even though he or she is compliant with a well-managed antipsychotic drug treatment program (Falloon et al. 1982).

Furthermore, more recent work has demonstrated that reducing this expressed hostility also reduces the relapse rate. It is important to understand that this is of no minor significance. For example, over a two-year period we may expect between a 20 and 40 percent relapse rate in schizophrenic patients adequately maintained on an antipsychotic drug treatment program. Effective attention to the emotional climate in which the patient exists seems to reduce this relapse rate to less than 10 percent. It is imperative, especially in the treatment of refractory or erratically responding patients, that the physician carefully attend to the overall emotional climate in which the patient lives.

The second issue is the process of recuperation. It is perhaps most fitting to close with a discussion of this issue because it brings us back to the basic interconnection of the psychosocial and the biological. Some evidence suggests that careful attention to the recuperative process is important in facilitating a good and lasting drug response. This means that a patient is more vulnerable to relapse from stressful situations or difficult undertakings during the period immediately after a drug-facilitated change versus after some time has elapsed and a lasting stabilization has been achieved. Findings supporting such a notion include Janowsky et al.'s (1973) work demonstrating the ease in eliciting schizophrenic symptoms in recovered schizophrenic patients via amphetamine stimulation soon after recovery, but not after recovery has been present for a longer period of time. Further support comes from findings of a high relapse rate with drug discontinuation immediately postrecovery, and a positive correlation between the degree of recovery obtained in the hospital and postdischarge time to relapse (Goldberg et al. 1977).

From a psychosocial perspective this suggests that the physician must carefully monitor how much stress the patient subjects himself or herself to after the initial response to drug treatment. The degree of stress and activity a patient undergoes must be carefully graduated and controlled. The physician must understand what the sources of real stress are in the patient's life. With which relatives is the patient likely to have a difficult interaction? What aspects of work are difficult for the patient to manage? Do any specific household tasks cause the patient more or less anxiety? What is the sum total of activities in which the patient engages that may lead him or her to feel overwhelmed? Another question for the patient who is not achieving recovery is whether the situation in which he or she lives is so stressful that partial movements toward recovery are continuously undermined by persisting psychosocial demands on the patient, and should the living situation be altered either by reducing activity level or via temporary hospitalization in order to support the recovery process?

In summary, by systematic attention to those psychosocial variables that influence medication compliance and facilitate or interfere with the development of the therapeutic alliance, those issues that may arise in psychotherapy to adversely or inappropriately influence the course of pharmacotherapy, and those psychosocial forces that influence the recovery process, more effective psychopharmacological treatment programs can be assured.

REFERENCES

Becker MH, Maiman LA: Strategies for enhancing compliance. J Community Health 6:113–135, 1980

Blackwell B: The drug regimen and treatment compliance, in Compliance in Health Care. Edited by Haynes RB, Taylor DW, Sackett DL. Baltimore, MD, Johns Hopkins University Press, 1979

Christensen DB: Drug-taking compliance: a review and synthesis. Health Serv Res 13:171–187, 1978

Docherty JP: Psychotherapy and pharmacotherapy: clinical problems. Yale Psychiatric Quarterly 00:2–11, 1979

Docherty JP, Fiester SJ: The therapeutic alliance and compliance with psychopharmacology, in Psychiatry Update, Annual Review (Vol 4). Edited by Hales R, Francis A. Washington, DC, American Psychiatric Press, 1985

Ettlinger PRA, Freedman GL: General practice compliance study: is it worth being a personal doctor? Br Med J 282:1192–1194, 1981

Evans L, Spelman M: The problem of noncompliance with drug therapy. Drugs 25:63–76, 1983

Falloon I, Boyd J, McGill CW, et al: Family management in the prevention of exacerbations of schizophrenia: a controlled study. N Engl J Med 306:1437–1440, 1982

Goldberg SC, Schooler NR, Hogarty GE, et al: Predictions of relapse in schizophrenic outpatients treated by drug and sociotherapy. Arch Gen Psychiatry 34:171–184, 1977

Gordis L: Conceptual and methodological problems in measuring patient compliance, in Compliance in Health Care. Edited by Haynes RB, Taylor DW, Sackett DL. Baltimore, MD, Johns Hopkins University Press, 1979

Hartley D: Research on the therapeutic alliance in psychotherapy, in Psychiatry Update, Annual Review (Vol 4). Edited by Hales R, Francis A. Washington, DC, American Psychiatric Press, 1985

Haynes RB: A critical review of the determinants of patient compliance with therapeutic regimens, in Compliance With Therapeutic Regimens. Edited by Sackett DL, Haynes RB. Baltimore, MD, Johns Hopkins University Press, 1976

Janowsky DS, El-Yousef MK, Davis JM, et al: Provocation of schizophrenic symptoms by intravenous administration of methylphenidate. Am J Psychiatry 28:185–191, 1973

Malahy B: The effect of instruction and labeling on the number of medication errors made by patients at home. Am J Hosp Pharm 23:283–292, 1966

Marston M: Compliance with medical regimens: a review of the literature. Nurs Res 19:312–323, 1970

Stimson GV: Obeying doctors' orders: a view form the other side. Soc Sci Med 8:97–104, 1974

VanPutten T: Drug refusal in schizophrenia: causes and prescribing units. Hosp Community Psychiatry 29:110–112, 1978

APPENDIX

Compliance Checklist

1. Presence, Form, and Degree of Noncompliance
   A. What is the type of noncompliance?
      Overdosing
      Underdosing
      Improper or erratic dosing
   B. What is the pattern of noncompliance?
      Missed doses
      Missed days
   C. What is the report of patient compliance?
      By relatives
      By pill count
      By structured interview

2. The Patient
   A. What are the patient's expressed reasons for
      noncompliance?
      Intelligent
      Capricious
      Refusal
      Confused
      Misdirection
   B. What is the patient's previous history of noncompliance?
   C. What does the patient believe of the illness?
      Does the patient believe that if he or she stops the medication
         the illness will return or worsen?
      Does the patient perceive the illness as serious
         and severe?
      Does the patient believe the treatment will be helpful?
      Does the patient perceive the treatment to be of undue finan-
         cial, social, psychological, or physical cost?
   D. Are there particular aspects of the illness that might affect
      compliance?
      Denial of the illness
      Cognitive disorganization
      History/presence of avoidance behavior
      Irrational beliefs

E. What is the current family and social situation?
Stability
Attitudes

3. Psychopharmacological Regimen
   A. What is the patient's tolerance for or compatibility with the side effects and associated properties of the drug?
      Sedation
      Other treatment emergent side effects
   B. What is the dosage schedule?
      Complexity
      Frequency
      Duration
   C. What degree of change is required in the patient's daily behavior?
      Change of diet
      Change of activity
      Change of sleep time
      Change of work schedule
   D. By what route is the medication administered?
   E. Cost

4. Physician–Patient Relationship
   A. Has the doctor been explicit in telling the patient what the patient must do to properly follow the treatment program?
   B. Have the patient and doctor clearly stated what each expects of the other in the treatment?
   C. Is the patient accepting responsibility for carrying out his or her part of the treatment?
   D. Is the tone of the relationship positive and supportive?

5. Overall Treatment Program and Setting
   A. Is there continuity in the patient care?
      Clinician
      Office setting
      Appointment time
   B. Is there interruption or irregularity in the treatment program?
      Missed/canceled appointments
      Long waiting time